MUSIC UNLIMITED

For Keith and Mary.

With all good wishes.

Yehudi

Kentner

Performing Arts Studies

A series of books edited by Janice Rieman

Volume 1
Music Unlimited
The Performer's Guide to New Audiences
Isabel Farrell and Kenton Mann

Additional volumes in preparation:

Inner Rhythm
Naomi Benari

Experimental Music Notebooks
Leigh Landy

This book is part of a series. The publisher will accept continuation orders which may be cancelled at any time and which provide for automatic billing and shipping of each title in the series upon publication. Please write for details.

MUSIC UNLIMITED

The Performer's Guide to New Audiences

Isabel Farrell and Kenton Mann

Faculty of Art and Design, Manchester Metropolitan University, UK

harwood academic publishers

Switzerland • Australia • Belgium • France • Germany • Great Britain
India • Japan • Malaysia • Netherlands • Russia • Singapore • USA

Harwood Academic Publishers

Private Bag 8
Camberwell, Victoria 3124
Australia

3-14-9, Okubo
Shinjuku-ku, Tokyo 169
Japan

12 Cour Saint-Eloi
75012 Paris
France

Emmaplein 5
1075AW Amsterdam
Netherlands

Christburger Strasse II
10405 Berlin
Germany

820 Town Center Drive
Langhorne, Pennsylvania 19047
United States of America

Post Office Box 90
Reading, Berkshire RG1 8JL
Great Britain

Library of Congress Cataloging-in-Publication Data

Farrell, Isabel, 1937-
    Music unlimited: the performer's guide to new audiences/Isabel
Farrell and Kenton Mann.
        p.   cm, — (Performing arts studies, ISSN 0891-6281: V. 1)
    Includes index.
    ISBN 3-7186-5525-X (hardback): $29.00. — ISBN 3-7186-5526-8
(softback): $14.00
    1. Music audiences. 2. Music — Performance.   3. Concerts.
I. Mann, Kenton, 1969- . II. Title. III. Series.
ML3795.F32 1994
780'. 78 — dc20   94-2405
                                                                         CIP
                                                                         MN

CONTENTS

INTRODUCTION TO THE SERIES

Performing Arts Studies aims to provide stimulating resource books of both a practical and philosophical nature for teachers and students of the performing arts: music, dance, theatre, film, radio, video, oral poetry, performance art, and multi-media forms.

International and multicultural in scope and content, Performing Arts Studies seeks to represent the best and most innovative contemporary directions in performing arts education, and will focus particularly on the work of practising artists who are also involved in teaching.

JANICE RIEMAN

Acknowledgements

This book would not have been possible without the help of many people.

The authors wish to thank:-

Margaret Archibald – the London Mozart Players
Sandy Broadhurst – Gorton Brook School, Manchester
Marjorie Dickenson – Oakdale School, Tameside
Clients and staff at the Jubilee Centre, Bolton
Sara Lee – Music Tutor, HMP Wormwood Scrubs
Sylvia Lindsay MBE – President Emeritus, The Council for Music in Hospitals
Margaret McLay and students – Chetham's School of Music
Richard McNicol –the Apollo Trust
Ann Morisy – The London Diocesan Board for Social Responsibility

for their invaluable contributions.

Thanks are also due to everyone who allowed us to quote them and use their photographs, to Lynn Davies – Assistant Director, Social Services, Salford, to Denise Clark for her indefatigable typing and to the Royal Northern College of Music, Manchester, UK, where it all began.

Prelude

"The changing wisdom of successive generations discards ideas, questions facts, demolishes theories. But the artist appeals to that part of our being which is not dependent on wisdom ... He speaks to our capacity for delight and wonder, to the sense of mystery surrounding our lives: to our sense of pity, and beauty, and pain; to the latent feeling of fellowship with all creation." (Joseph Conrad)

In every city, town and village, there are people who are denied the opportunity to hear live music. They live in remote rural areas, or places where the last bus home goes at 8 o'clock. They are spending their lives in hospitals, prisons and innumerable other institutions. They are wheelchair users lacking access to many public buildings and underprivileged children in inner cities.

All of these people are potential audiences for music groups who will take the trouble to seek them out. This book is designed to be a performer's companion – informing your decisions as you prepare performances. With the help of colleagues, we describe some of the situations in which you will find yourselves, and also the techniques which work for us while performing in community venues.

The value to your audience is in the excitement, the aural and visual stimulation, the educational content and the enormous amount of sheer fun that your performance will provide. The response from a community audience is immediate and unfeigned. You will discover straight away that community performances are the quickest possible learning process. You will find your performances stimulating and confidence building. You will learn to think on your feet, to improvise and to respond instantly to the needs of your audience. One such performance will teach you more about yourselves and your playing than you can learn in a whole year on the concert circuit. As you enrich other people's lives, so will your own lives also be enriched.

Have courage. So long as you care deeply about what you are doing, there are millions of ways to do it right.

Preparation

"I believe in Michael Angelo, Velasquez and Rembrandt; in the might of design; the mystery of color, the redemption of all things by Beauty everlasting, and the message of Art that has made these hands blessed."
(George Bernard Shaw)

The scope for concerts in community venues is unlimited. Lack of understanding, ignorance, fear of the unknown – all inhibit musicians from taking the first steps towards hugely exciting and rewarding experiences. Our aim is to give you information and insight so that you can take those first steps with confidence.

To write a book of this kind generalizations have to be made. Be aware that each individual venue is unique. You cannot take *anything* for granted.

Programme planning lies at the heart of your preparation. It is the music you produce which makes you special. We discuss presentation techniques and "preparing the listening", but these are mere tools used to attract and emphasise. It is the quality of the music and the quality of your playing which is paramount.

Why then do you need this book? Why are practise and rehearsal on their own, not enough? You have in your skills and techniques a unique means of communication – unique, but not infallible.

Consider the context in which your performance will occur:-

For a performance in a concert hall, the audience has bought tickets on the strength of liking your published programme and wanting to hear you playing it. To achieve a satisfying experience for this audience, all you have to do is to turn up on time and play well.

The audience in a community venue, however, is very unlikely to have heard of you or your music. They may not even have been consulted as to whether they would like to listen to you or not. In

1

most cases, hospital staff, teachers, officers–in–charge will have made that decision for them. The concert hall audience has *chosen* to listen to you. The community audience has not necessarily been given that choice.

It is important that you realise the implication here because it radically changes your role – from a star performer to that of an outsider. In a community venue you are, essentially, a visitor. As such you will find that, to start with at any rate, the audience will be much more interested in you – your name, where you live etc. – than what you consider more important, your music.

Pre–Concert Visit

We strongly recommend that you visit each concert venue well in advance of the performance, in order to:–

1.   Meet your audience

It is enormously helpful to talk to an audience well ahead of the concert, when you are free from the pressures of performance. You won't have time to get to know each individual, but you will be able to talk to enough people to get a "feel" for the organisation. Read notice boards. Admire work on display. Get acquainted with the everyday life your audience leads.

In each venue you will notice that different titles are used. Some schools may refer to "children". Others will say "pupils" or "students". Adults may be referred to as "clients", "members" or "residents". Pick this up straight away, and use whichever title is recognised by the particular organisation. The courtesy will be appreciated.

Find out how many there will be in the audience. For a small group (under 30) you can plan a very relaxed, intimate concert. A larger audience may need a more formal approach.

2.   Assess the performance space

Seeing your performance space in advance can really make the difference between success and failure. There will be no back–up system of any kind, so take everything you could possibly need with you. Seating, lighting, audience arrangement, entrances, exits and the amount of room you have to play in – all have to be checked by you.

There is unlikely to be a raised performance area, so plan how the audience will see you best. Wheel chairs and high backed easy chairs are hard to see over and will need to be staggered if their occupants are to get a good view.

The performance space may be a school hall, a dining area, sitting room or recreation area. Whatever it is, make the most of it. To maximise the sight lines, seat the audience in the largest semicircle that will fit into the space and site yourselves in the middle of the semicircle. Place at least one aisle in the seating (if possible two or three) so that you can easily move around the audience. Don't play with your back to the light and, since doorways may be in use during the concert, station yourselves as far from them as possible. If you need to bring extra lighting with you, check the wall sockets.

3.   Preparing the listening

The best compliment that any audience can pay you is the quiet concentration of positive listening. Listening (hearing *plus* attention) is a skill that, like any other, needs to be practised. Your audience may not be practised listeners.

As experienced musicians, it is easy to take our listening skills and aural training for granted. What we consider obvious (changes of timbre and texture, counterpoint etc.) may be nothing of the sort to an untrained ear. Recall your own experience with other art forms. A magazine article or television documentary can transform the way you look at a painting. You perceive the painting in a completely different way when you understand more about the artist's aims and techniques. Your "looking" has been prepared. So it will be with your audience and their listening.

Take time to consider your appearance. Day time gigs, draughty halls, stuffy day rooms, will all influence the way you dress. Don't underestimate the effect of looking "special". If you are worth looking at, you will be worth listening to.

Programme notes are the accepted way in which an audience is informed about the music they are going to hear. For a number of reasons, a printed programme in this area of work is unlikely to be appropriate. Your programme notes will be delivered in a spoken introduction. The introductions will give listening cues and, even more important, convey your own enthusiasm for the music. This personal contact with the music you are going to play is invaluable, and promotes sympathetic listening.

The prospect of speaking to an audience can be daunting. As ever, practice will make perfect. Bear the following in mind:–

* *Prepare what you are going to say.* In rehearsal, it is so easy to spend two hours on the sixth bar after B, and five minutes on the introductions while packing away. Your introductions are part of the "thread". They weld a collection of pieces into a complete musical experience. Design your spoken introductions with the same care that you put into rehearsing the music.

* *Don't rush.* When the adrenalin is flowing, we tend to speak too quickly. Pacing an introduction will develop with experience. In the mean time, speak clearly and just keep it steady. Wait for applause and audience buzz to die down before starting to speak.

* *Be yourself.* There is no need to put on an act. Any form of insincerity immediately communicates itself to an audience and they will resent it. Don't worry too much about suitable vocabulary. You will find that you automatically adjust the way you relay information to your listeners, according to their age. For instance – a group of potential sponsors may be just as interested in the way an octave key works as a group of nursery children, but the tone of your presentation to each group will be different.

* *Your introduction must be relevant.* It is important to give each of music its proper title and to name its composer, but talking about dates/2nd subject/ritornello etc., will do very little in themselves to prepare an untrained ear. A personal approach is far more effective.

* *Introduce yourselves by name.* Talk about yourselves – how long you have been playing together, where you live, where you rehearse, why you like working together. Tell your audience what it is about a particular piece of music that appeals to you; why you included it in the programme; which instrument has the tune/the difficult bit/a major solo. Give people things to listen out for – dynamics, instrumentation, rhythm patterns, etc. By controlling the audience's expectation you enhance their concentration.

* *There will always be interest in your instruments* – how they work, what they are made of, how much they cost, and why you like to play them. Encourage questions and make sure everyone has a close-up view. If you use any unfamiliar term (reed, bow, mouthpiece) explain it as you go along. Don't forget – one demonstration is worth a ton of explanation. Properly thought out and integrated demonstrations will keep the "thread" of your performance intact, and encourage concentration at the same time.

* *Support the speaker.* While he is speaking, get his next piece ready for him. Listen to what he is saying and look at him. This is crucial with younger audiences – if *you* don't listen neither will they. If he needs props, have them ready. If he laughs, you laugh. If he dries, look supportive! and fill in for him. In our experience, this type of team approach always leads to a tighter and more sensitive ensemble.

* Always acknowledge applause – together.

Concentration is often at a premium in community venues. Learning difficulties, sensory impairment, illness, the hubbub of institutional life, can all affect the length and depth of an audience's concentration.

With this in mind, you should first establish the length of the performance and agree with the venue appropriate times to begin (and end) your performance. Starting and finishing times are critical. All institutions work to the clock – the larger the institution, the less flexible it is.

Starting times ought to be a case of contractual obligation. Stop times may not be so clear cut. Discuss the duration with staff and find out what will happen immediately after your performance. Five minutes too long, and your audience may disappear during your finale – too short and you may find yourself suffering "death by encores". Careful planning will keep you in control.

Having established the duration of your programme (typically, one hour without an interval) the content can be finalised. Different groups will have diverse challenges at this stage. A string quartet could easily fill an hour with three works, but push the audience beyond its concentration span. A quartet of trombones might need a dozen pieces to fill the same time, which could easily become a list, rather than a programme.

What is required is a sense of "balance" – not just how long is a piece, but where it should come in the programme? What demands does it make on the listener? How does this piece affect those around it?

As performers, this process is normally controlled for us by the composer. If you are playing a Brahms symphony, it is Brahms who controls the listener's expectations and emotions as the work unfolds. Each movement has its own mood, yet it is part of a balanced whole. The Adagietto from Mahler's 5th is often heard on its own, but playing it anywhere else *within the symphony* would be unthinkable.

We call this factor the "emotional thread", and in your concert the thread will be very much in your hands.

Two Sample Programmes

The Kreutzer Quartet – Peter Shepherd and Clio Gould (violins), Philip Dukes (viola) and Philip Shepherd (cello) rehearse a different core repertoire for each year.

In 1990 this core repertoire was

Haydn	Quartet Op 64, No 4.
Sibelius	Quartet "Voces Intimae" Op 56.
Bartok	Quartet No. 3 (1927).
Puccini	Elegy (Chrysanthemums).
Mozart	Divertimento K136.

They plan every programme for the year – from major recitals to performances for community audiences – juggling pieces from the repertoire to make a suitable programme for each event. They will also use other pieces already in their repertoire.

For instance – one programme for community audiences, planned to show how stringed instruments work and the relationship between them, began with extracts from the Bach Double Violin Concerto and included two Roumanian Dances as well as the last movement of the Bartok Quartet; the final movement of the Haydn; Britten's "Playful Pizzicato"; a solo viola version of "Happy Birthday" and, as an encore, an original arrangement of "If You Knew Suzie".

The Trombone Quartet, Bone Idols – Anthony Howe, Robert Holliday, Jason Glover and Paul Milner – recently performed a programme designed to show contrasts in musical effects:–

Duke Ellington	Caravan
Flor Peters	Suite (3rd Movement)
Schumann	Traumerei
Gareth Wood	Four Pieces for Four Trombones (4th Movement)
Flor Peters	Suite (1st Movement)
Bruckner	Locus Iste
Joplin	Cascades
Delibes	Pizzicato
Jerome Kern	All The Things You Are.

Only you can visualise the way your programme will balance. Assuming you already have considerable experience and a core repertoire, you must play music to which you are committed. The following points, however, will be relevant to any performance.

A) Your first piece is vitally important. Given the extra–musical factors mentioned earlier, you may well have to start stone cold. Your opening music must seize the attention of the audience and set the atmosphere you want. If the piece does not exist, write or arrange one. A collection of "openers", each invoking a different atmosphere, is invaluable.

B) With the concept of the "emotional thread" on board, each piece you play will be placed to optimise its effect on your audience. Listen to each piece through the ears of the audience. As the programme unfolds, so you establish a framework for listening. Don't let other factors get in the way. You may, for instance, wish to programme an experimental and challenging work. If you use criteria such as stamina, rather than programme balance, the work may come too soon, receive a confused hearing and concentration may fragment. Concentration is a precious commodity. It links the audience with the thread of your performance.

C) Although the clock may decide *when* you finish, you can determine *how* you finish. The last piece rounds off the proceedings and careful choice can avoid the "is that it?" syndrome. It is worth building some flexibility into the last part of your programme so that you can ensure that you do finish with your chosen "finisher".

Get close to your audience – as close as practicable. If your audience are close enough to see valves/keys/fingers working, this visual contact will support the listening.

Music stands can be an iron curtain when it comes to communication. As musicians we feel secure sitting down behind a stand. We do our job – playing the notes – someone else does the P.R. This is not an option for community audiences. Demonstration and introductions should be performed in front of the stands. Busking and improvisation are ways of exploiting the "feel" of your instrument. When you are close to a 'cello, tuba or piano, you can feel as well as hear it. Take along old instruments or mock–ups so people can actually touch a vibrating string or pipe. The one–to–one element will be appreciated by any audience and, for those with aural or visual impairment, the moment can be exquisite.

Following Up Your Performance

A thank you letter to the person who booked you is obviously good business practice. Your letter, displayed or read out, will be appreciated by all those who were involved. Recollections of your performance may spark off discussions, workshops or other art work. In remembering, people will then look forward to your next visit. In institutional life, the value of having something to look forward to cannot be over–stated.

Ask people to send you feed–back of any description. Paintings, letters, photographs are all intrinsically valuable. They are also evidence of success when you approach other venues or make bids for funding.

A portfolio of audience criticism and appreciation is a powerful publicity tool, with just as much potential as your most flattering press clippings. Cultivate it carefully.

Develop links with venues where you have made friends and built trust. As a friend you will be in a strong position to encourage people to come to your public concerts. Many orchestras in the UK (Halle, BBC Philharmonic etc.) have successfully fostered access in this way. There is no reason why your ensemble cannot be part of this very important and deeply rewarding process.

Concerts for Schools' Audiences

"If you stimulate a body, that body will learn." (anon.)

Schools vary enormously in size and atmosphere according to their geographical location and a host of other factors. Don't assume that the school at which you are going to perform will be at all the same as the ones you went to yourself. Go to see it, and find out. The rural primary school, for instance, presents you with an entirely different audience to that in a large city high school.

The crucial factor in planning music for children and young people is to cater for the right age range. Remember the difference in attitudes and perceptions between you as a five year old and you as a teenager. Liaise with staff – not only the Head and the music teacher, but also the class teachers of the children for whom you will perform. The number and age range of your audience needs to be confirmed in writing well in advance of your concert date.

Your Audience

Primary schools (5–11 year olds)

Concerts in primary schools are welcomed by the staff, who will want as many children as possible to benefit from taking part. Until you are experienced, resist the suggestion that the whole school sit on the floor of the school hall to listen to you. Roughly speaking, the younger the children in the audience, the smaller the audience should be. Very young children have a short attention span and, by the time a large number get settled, their capacity for good behaviour may be quite exhausted. You, and your audience, will get more out of the performance if you play for smaller groups in the informal surroundings of their own classrooms.

Working with a small group, you can quickly get on a first name basis. Everyone can be allowed to touch the instruments and/or ask questions. You can sit in the middle of the class with children watching closely how you play. You will have the time to notice individual reactions and to respond to them.

The children will want to be part of your performance. Plan the programme to give them the opportunity to discuss mood, textures, height and depth of sound, likes and dislikes. Play all the different sounds of which your instrument is capable, and finish with something in which everyone can join.

High schools (12–16 year olds)

For very many young people the only music to which they have access is of the "canned" variety. Music is something which you switch on when you want it. Most teenagers will have little idea of the effort, time and energy that must be expended on producing it, and no concept at all of the enormous range of music that is available. The 13 – 15 age group can be difficult to enthuse and involve, but you will find that everyone responds to quality and honesty of performance.

One way of breaking the ice is to visit your prospective audience and involve them in a discussion on a music–related subject – how to go about making music a career; earning your living as a free–lance musician; any other relevant topic about which you are well–informed and/or feel strongly. If you have the opportunity to do this, your audience will approach the coming performance in an entirely different frame of mind, and will be listening to your music as the work of a friend, not as something which the Powers That Be think is good for them.

Special schools

The phrase "with learning difficulties" covers those children who, for a variety of reasons, are regarded as unable to take advantage of mainstream education. The present trend in the U.K., is to integrate pupils with learning difficulties into main–stream education, but plenty of special schools still exist – many of them having strong links with a neighbouring main–stream school.

Special schools cater for children with moderate, severe and complex learning difficulties. The age ranges may be comparable with those in main stream schools, but some special schools have pupils whose ages range from 3 – 18 years. Teachers have many special skills and will often be assisted by other care staff.

Among pupils attending special schools you can expect to find those with a very short attention span, those who are emotionally unstable and those who are hyperactive. There may also be contributary physical factors. There will be pupils with severely limited communication skills, combined with profound movement difficulties, in almost any combination.

Special educational establishments also exist for pupils with visual handicaps, for those with speech problems and for those with very poor hearing.

Obviously, children with disabilities may fit into more than one of the above categories. It is not safe to assume that all the pupils at a school for children with a hearing impairment will have *only* the problem of deafness with which to contend.

In preparing a performance for an audience in a special school, a pre-concert visit to the school is *essential*. Spend as much time as you can talking to children and staff and use the information you acquire to plan your programme. When addressing and motivating children, take your cue from the staff and go along with the behaviour they demonstrate as appropriate.

The immediate attraction of live music makes it an ideal medium for communication. Concerts provide opportunities for learning by creating the kind of stimuli which can help pupils achieve the hitherto unachieveable.

Throughout your programme BE AWARE of children who are nervous, either of you or of loud sounds; of children with hearing aids – instruments played too close can cause actual pain; of children who know all the answers and are dying to join in (often on the back row). Always acknowledge applause – extravagantly.

Amongst all your audiences it will be obvious to you that there are children with limited motor skills. Don't let this inhibit you from carrying out a programme which includes physical response. If properly briefed by you, staff will assist the less able, and everyone will benefit from trying. Some children will astonish you by their level of achievement and enjoyment.

"There really is something special about live music. James is a profoundly handicapped child with very little sight and poor hearing. Positive responses from James are rare indeed. What could be nicer than to see this child responding to the sound of the clarinets. Perhaps it is only those who know him well who could fully appreciate his reactions. He was moving his head to where the sound was coming from and, when we put his hands round the instrument as it was played, he smiled."
(Birtle View School, Rochdale.)

Over and over again, we have had experience of individual children most happily joining in with everything that is going on, only to find out later that these children have never made a positive response to *any* classroom experience before.

You will, necessarily, have only a short aquaintance with the pupils for whom you are performing. You cannot be aware of every child's abilities and, even though you will be much applauded, will not be able to assess fully the effect of your playing. The reaction from members of your audience may be overwhelming, or minimal; it may be what you expect – or totally unexpected.

* *

From Sandy Broadhurst, Gorton Brook School, Manchester.

""Miss! Miss! Wasn't it great yesterday? When can we go again?"

This has been the inevitable response when, over the years, I have taken children to listen to live music. Whatever the kind of music and however unfamiliar to the children, they have always reacted positively. The magic of wonderful music, coming almost from nowhere, from a variety of weird shaped instruments, big, little, shiny, dull, visually exciting in themselves, *never* ceases to reach children.

Music, somehow, has the ability to reach across the barriers of intelligence, poverty and culture and touch children, enriching their lives and bringing joy to often grey worlds. Even years later, I have had children say to me, "Do you remember, Miss, when you took us to ...." These musical experiences have become part of a wealth of childhood memories.

When children leave school, if they never read another book or write another sentence, we can be sure they will still hear music. It is a part of all our lives – the T.V. 'ads', background music in plays and 'soaps', film scores, Top of the Pops, ... music is everywhere around us. Helping children to listen and interpret and be aware of this music, adds an extra depth and dimension to their lives. We can listen to music on tape or record but *nothing* replaces the magic of listening to music played live.

Music also plays a vital part in helping children with learning difficulties to develop various skills, particularly those associated with reading. Poorly developed attention and listening skills, and problems with auditory discrimination and memory are often underlying causes of children failing to learn. Music offers a stimulating and fun way of helping these skills to develop.

'Listen ... am I playing fast or slow?'
'Listen ... am I playing loudly or quietly?'
'Listen ... am I playing high or low?'

'Listen, I'm going to play loudly, when I change to play quietly put up your hand.'

'I'm going to play a tune ... now we're going to play together ... when you hear the special tune put up your hand.'

The possibilities are endless. Because the situation is exciting and different, children are highly motivated and so they learn. They extend their powers of attention and concentration and acquire the ability to discriminate sounds. They develop not only musical skills but vital pre-reading skills as well.

Just think, all this *and* the magic of live music too.

The links between poverty and poor educational achievement are well documented. This connection can clearly be seen in the field of musical education. Because of poverty many parents from inner city areas are unable to take their children to hear the rich variety of music available locally. Children are thus denied a vital musical experience. 'Live Music Now' helps to overcome this problem by providing concerts free and so making live music accessible to all children.

Education has variously been described as 'an encounter with excellence' and 'an initiation into worthwhile activities'. 'Live Music Now', which helps to develop vital learning skills, gives children an insight and extra perspective to their lives and brings joy and magic into their world, is certainly both of these things. It is education in its fullest sense. On behalf of many children with learning difficulties, who have gained great happiness through its work, thank you.

From Mrs. A. A. Shaw, NNEB Course Tutor, North Cheshire College.

"Thank you very much for having my Nursery Nursing students to the Chione Trio Concert for children with special needs.

As well as enjoying the music, the afternoon turned out to be a most stimulating learning experience for the students, in seeing how children, with a wide range of disabilities, responded so spontaneously and with such obvious enjoyment to the music. We were very interested to observe how quickly the children became involved and how well they participated.

We agreed that the programme was very well planned and balanced to the children's interests and span of attention."

From Mrs. Lisa M. Howarth, Head Tacher, Birtle View School, Heywood.

""Phoenix Brass were fantastic!!   Phoenix Brass ARE fantastic!!

Without exception the staff were delighted with the way in which our children responded to their playing, their sensitivity and their humour. Their visit will be long remembered as a highlight in our school year.

On behalf of the children, their parents and the staff may I thank you for sponsoring the input we received.   I know that the quintet are professionally very busy, but, so great was their impact that I would like to re-book them at some time in the future.

I enclose some comments from our children which I hope you will enjoy looking at, but, by far the greatest privilege was to be here and witness the effect, particularly on those of our children who experience profound and multiple handicaps and who cannot formally record their appreciation."

Adults With Learning Difficulties

"Art is not a handicraft, it is the transmission of feeling the artist has experienced." (Leo Tolstoy)

On leaving special school at 16–19 a person unable to take advantage of mainstream training or employment will probably be offered a place in an Adult Training Centre.

Originally set up to offer clients an occupation – sorting, packing, laundry work – the need for personal and social education programmes is now widely recognised.

Moves are now being made to integrate clients into their community and to break down the insularity of the A.T.C. Some authorities call their establishments Social Education Centres. These centres function as a base from which clients can access education, training and the arts, including live music. There are, however, many traditional A.T.C's, without the resources to travel, who would warmly welcome a live performance being brought to them.

Working With the Staff

A.T.C.'s are run by the local social services, not by education authorities. Staff therefore work an industrial year with far fewer holidays than education establishments.

Music specialists are rare in A.T.C.'s, so staff are likely to be very enthusiastic about your input. One concert will not change a client's life but it can provide staff with valuable spin–off material. A concert can be looked forward to, experienced and so, so important, REMEMBERED.

Although your first contact will be with the Manager or Deputy Manager, before (and during) your performance you will be liaising with Centre Officers and Care Staff. Try and find out exactly which staff will be present at your performance. Take some time to share ideas and experiences. Do not assume that senior staff will brief them on what you intend to do or what you might expect of them; far better to do it yourself.

Your Audience

It is hard to imagine an audience more diverse and complex. In terms of age, experience and understanding the difference from client to client can be enormous. The question "what should we play?" just does not arise. Simply perform music to which you are committed, whilst bearing in mind the following points.

1. First impressions can be misleading. You may not know until after the performance just how successful you were. Staff will often point out clients who showed new behaviour or reactions whilst you were playing. A major achievement may be so easily missed whilst playing, or just accepted as the norm.

2. People with learning difficulties can easily become confused. The daily routine into which you will step provides clients with a sense of security and purpose. Many clients will derive motivation and self-esteem from their daily tasks. What may appear work-a-day or even trivial could, in fact, be a central part of someone's day. Your performance needs to be an enrichment of, not a disruption to, the daily pattern. Knowing this will inform your discussions with staff and help you to cope with things that might arise during your performance.

3. Some clients, particularly in their late teens and early twenties, may not have had the opportunity to develop social skills. You must be prepared for clients to respond with their "essence" – swaying, shouting, clapping, as an accompaniment to your playing. People can only learn appropriate behaviour as a result of experience. When live music becomes part of the life of an A.T.C., then listening skills will become part of a client's repertoire.

4. The sense of occasion which your performance will generate is infectious and a highly rewarding aspect of the job. *Music will have strong associations in your audience's mind.* Whilst they may not be seasoned concert goers, music is a regular feature of social activity. Add to this the excitement of your visit and you have a bubbling atmosphere. Controlling the enthusiasm and channeling the energy into listening is the key to success. (See Preparing the Listening in the chapter "Preparation".)

    Playing serious, unfamiliar works takes courage, but why not? Quality, rhythmic energy, sonority can appeal across any barrier. There is nothing wrong with playing tunes which people know, but there is nothing like the quality of experience which can be shared when new sounds and textures are discovered. Do not be afraid of failure. In A.T.C.'s the word does not exist.

From Garry Jackson, Wythenshawe Adult Training Centre

"The audience reaction was surprisingly positive considering that most people's access to classical music is very limited. The calm content of some of the pieces balanced against lively folk music (Bartok) worked well.

The relationship between the violins, viola and cello was explained, as was their roles in the various pieces played, and this was well understood.

The programme (50 minutes) could easily have been longer. It was planned on the assumption of a short concentration span but, if the works performed differ in tempo, mood and style, this really shouldn't be a problem. However, it was the first time we have had music of this nature and it is too easy to be knowledgeable with hindsight.

All who heard the programme wanted to know when the musicians were coming again."

From Vivienne Hancox, Orchard Mount, Eccles, Manchester

"For the person with learning difficulties, live music gives an opportunity for creativity and achievement. Music can be made and enjoyed, however limited the involvement or the understanding.

Taking part in live music can be an exciting, sensitive time, where feelings are easily expressed. Above all, it is fun!"

People Who Attend Rehabilitation and Resource Centres

"Life without industry is guilt, and industry without art is brutality."
(John Ruskin)

Rehabilitation Centres are run by the local Health Authority and exist for people who, usually as a result of illness or accident, have partially or completely lost a skill necessary to their normal lives. The patients mostly live in their own homes and, in order to re–learn lost skills, attend the centre for anything from one to five days a week.

It is possible to learn a huge range of different skills at the centre – everything from speech therapy to cooking or how to wash your hair – so a large number of staff with specialised skills will direct sessions on a very strict timetable. This may make the timing of your performance difficult, though there will often be one afternoon a week when efforts are made to provide leisure activities. Many staff feel that it is important to have an occasion on which everyone can meet together and enjoy themselves.

Resource Centres are run by Social Services and cater for people who have physical disabilities and who are unable to be employed. The clients, who may live either at home or in a hostel, attend daily – Monday to Friday – and there will sometimes be evening activities as well. Since the resources available reflect as far as possible the wishes and needs of the clients, they vary, but will often include sports and leisure activities, crafts and library facilities.

Your Audience

At both Resource and Rehabilitation Centres your audience will be people aged 18 and over with some physical problems. Your first contact will be with either the Sister in Charge (Rehabilitation Centres) or the Officer in Charge (Resource Centres) whom you do need to meet well ahead of the concert.

Some Centres will plan leisure activities with the co-operation of their clients. In others the staff may decide (for whatever reason) that a concert is a good idea, without reference to those who are going to be listening to it. These varying approaches make a huge difference to the way in which your audience will regard you. Most will welcome you unreservedly but, if they feel "put upon" or patronised you may well find it very hard work and an uphill struggle to establish lines of communication.

A preliminary visit to the Centre beforehand should sort out most of these problems, especially if you make an opportunity to talk to your prospective audience. If you do meet resentment, or even anger, try to remember that it is not aimed at you, but at the world in general.

At some Resource Centres there may be a hearing impaired group in the audience. The staff will feel, quite rightly, that this group should be included in every activity. The problem this can cause at a concert is noisy interruptions by people who are not aware of the noise they are making. The rest of the audience will pay no attention because they will be used to it – so you will have to take it in your stride as well.

Your Performance

The members of your audience may, as a result of their awareness of their limited abilities, have low self-esteem. However much they appreciate your programme and your playing, they are unlikely to be enthusiastic straight away and will take time to warm up. This is a prime example of an occasion when you must not assume that the audience reaction isn't happening just because you don't immediately experience it.

Make your programme representative of many styles and moods of music and, in between performing, explain why you have chosen each piece. Your audience will be just as interested in you as in the music, so talk about yourselves – who you are, where you come from, why you chose to make music a career, why you like playing together/performing and especially all the awful/funny things that have happened to you as a group. Talk about your instruments and change the focus of attention by switching from playing to talking, to practical demonstrations. Make your playing interesting to watch as well as to hear.

* *

From The Report on The Jubilee Project by The Bolton Arts Unit, April, 1992.

Live Music Now! had been introduced to the Jubilee Centre, a day centre for people with physical disabilities in 1989 by the Social Services Department's Community Development Officer, and strong links were formed between the two organisations.

On 9th January 1992, work began on a major piece of music theatre. A total of thirteen workshops, lasting all day, took place over the next three months. All workshops were led by either a professional drama worker or one or more professional musicians. A storyline for a short piece of theatre was devised from the experiences of those taking part, eventually scripted, rehearsed and learnt. A song was written by the participants which celebrated the fellowship of the Jubilee Centre, and accompaniment to this was devised and rehearsed. The Apollo Saxophone quartet composed incidental music to accompany the dramatic action throughout the performance. A title for the production, "A Horse Designed by a Committee" was determined.

The first performance took place on the afternoon of 2nd April in front of a packed crowd at the Jubilee Centre. The production dealt with many of the realities of life for both disabled and able-bodied people and was greeted with acclaim by those who saw it. A cast of eleven formed the acting company, and the playing of the Apollo Saxophone quartet was augmented by an eleven strong group of musicians/singers from the Jubilee Centre.

Subsequent performances took place before an 80% house in the Octopus Studio of the Octagon Theatre in Bolton, and to smaller audiences at the Bury Metropolitan and at the Brickhouse Studio, Contact Theatre, Manchester. All those who saw the production expressed their enjoyment of the high standards of the production as well as gaining considerable amusement from some of the incidents in the storyline.

Any complex project of this nature has a wide number of benefits and spin-offs.

Through observation and discussion with the participants, it is evident that the following benefits accrued to participants: co-operation skills between participants increased; language skills increased alongside a greater ease in expressing conceptual ideas; participants were given confidence and their self-esteem was raised through the activity and they were better able to project that confidence; motor skills were developed; participants were given new status, particularly within their families; new skills in the creative arts

– both drama and music – were learnt by the participants; skills in development of creative work were increased. The participants experienced a sense of real achievement.

Through observation and discussion with the staff of the Jubilee Centre it is evident that the following benefits accrued to staff: rehabilitation staff were involved in the project as observers and internalised a great deal of the practice, leading to changes in their own practice, and also gave active support to the project, particularly through assistance in the making of scenery for the production and the construction of the wooden ramp for the Octagon; care staff saw participants in new roles within the activity, and became more aware of the potential within the participants and other centre users.

From Barbara Henderson, Manager, Jubilee Centre

"Last night was the last performance at Manchester of our current project.

I now know that the project presented the Centre users with a great challenge. In the beginning they had some reservations about the worthwhileness of such an event. Their own low self-esteem didn't allow them to realise or visualise how it could be.

As the play emerged and became almost a satire on themselves, their confidence began to build. One lady told me she felt less of a vegetable and became more of a person in her own right. All of the participants are discussing their new found self-confidence. Being coached by professional musicians seemed to speed up the performance level. They had an immediate standard to aspire to, rather than wandering around striving for an undefined level. They were able to identify more easily when they reached the "good enough" standard. They enjoyed writing the lyrics to the songs etc. Ed from the Education Department became their mainstay and the depth of commitment he had was amazing.

The result for the clients has been that they have gained in confidence, self-esteem, become people in their own right again, and gained status within their immediate family circle. I think this aspect has been the bonus, and perhaps one not always recognised by those of us fortunate enough to be able-bodied."

From Dusty Miller, Jubilee Centre, Bolton

"To Isabel and Sponsors of Jubilee Project.

This was one of the best things for all of us here at the Jubilee and I feel a lot has been learnt by us all.

We have benefited by working along side such well-qualified musicians, and learnt much. It will be experience put to good sense. I feel that not only should we explore the music side, but develop the role of the singers, in order that everyone participate to their maximum potential. I myself worked for many years in showbiz, I know my job well, 35 years of know how!, but still happy to learn new ideas and skills.

We all have or got a new vocation to go on. So please may I thank one and all. God Bless you, "Apollo", and all the sponsors. Thank you from our hearts."

Patients in Hospitals and Hospices

"The city is built to music, therefore never built at all, and therefore built forever." (Tennyson)

At the risk of underlining the obvious, it is important to remember that staff in hospitals are *busy*. Your music cannot be the most important thing that is going on. Priorities in hospitals will always be the physical well–being of the patients.

Since hospitals use a 24–hour timetable, shift work is inescapable. It is vital to keep this in mind when arranging performances. Find out which members of staff will be present for your performance. Make sure they realise that you want to perform for them as well as the patients, and that you value their opinions and input.

When making your pre–concert visit, leave a written reminder on the staff (or Ward) notice board, of the date and time, with your name and telephone number. If this can take the form of an attractive small leaflet, so much the better.

Your performing space may be anywhere and will almost certainly be part of a working area, in which case the privacy and dignity of the patients should be your first concern.

It may not be possible for your audience to be seated in a traditional manner, so you must make your performance mobile. You could play two or three pieces in different parts of the ward, and play a finale in the middle. It will be extremely helpful to be able to improvise and to have some music from memory.

Timing is important. Afternoon and early evening concerts will usually be best. Visiting times for relations are often unrestricted at weekends so you will be more welcome in mid–week. Exceptions to these general guidelines are some Hospices who like to have performances for patients *and* relatives/visitors, so that they can share the experience together.

* *

From Sylvia Lyndsay, MBE, President Emeritus, The Council for Music in Hospitals

I welcome the opportunity to share my thoughts on the value of live musical performances for people with the widely differing illnesses and disabilities whom we encounter in the hospitals; on the challenges, problems and rewards which the artist may encounter and the many skills needed in order to be able to give a successful hospital concert.

The venue in which you will be working may be a vast draughty hall, the social centre, a tea bar, a chapel, a tiny day room or by an individual bedside. In every case the success of the concert will be in direct relation to the ability of the artist to relate to the patients and to provide a suitable and extremely flexible programme.

I feel it is important that artists who are aiming to work in this field should understand something of the abilities and disabilities of a hospital audience in order to be able to assess their needs and adapt the programme and presentation accordingly.

Psychiatric Hospitals

The Council For Music in Hospitals was founded more than forty years ago and the first concerts were given in the large psychiatric hospitals. A large number of concerts are still given for these patients, who may be in hospital for a relatively short stay and then move on to rehabilitation centres, and later still will be found attending drop-in centres, or possibly living in hostels.

Patients may have bizarre thoughts and behaviour patterns and powerful mood swings. They may be suffering from clinical depression, sleeplessness or an overwhelming sensation of guilt, together with a feeling of their own worthlessness. In such places as Broadmoor and Ashworth (the secure hospitals) we also meet the profound personality disorders which produce extreme antisocial behaviour.

An understanding of these problems will prepare the musicians for finding an audience which may have a disruptive element. Many will be unable to sit through a concert – they will need to wander around, visit the loo, and some people will smoke incessantly. The use of drugs in their treatment can make them seem far away and apathetic in their responses, which can be worrying for a musician, who could be unaware that this is through no fault in the performance.

In addition to getting no response, there may be inappropriate reactions and this also is unnerving for an inexperienced performer. You must be prepared for laughter, tears or an hysterical outburst, all of which can in fact be of great value to the patient and may bring the long—awaited release of pent—up emotions enabling doctors and counsellors to approach and treat that particular patient.

A large proportion of the population in psychiatric hospitals now consists of elderly people who have been in hospital for many years suffering either from chronic mental illness or merely from a confused state of mind caused by their age. Remember that hospitals are home for such patients and concerts are an important means of bringing the outside world into the hospitals and of enriching the patients' lives.

The reports which we receive after each concert enable us to assess many of the benefits which our music brings to mentally ill patients. Staff comment on the high degree of interaction between the artists and their audience and tell us that patients seem to come to life and are different people when they are animated and enjoying an event of this kind. The happy atmosphere which is produced and the boost to morale of everyone concerned can linger for a long while after the music has finished. Meanwhile the doctors have gained a valuable insight into what can be achieved by this kind of therapeutic experience. Attending concerts can be a useful part of a rehabilitation programme and a preparation for going out into the word and learning to interact with those around them.

Frequently we hear of patients who talk for the first time for months and who will then be able to discuss their fears and their problems with the staff, or even with the artists, after the concert. It is sometimes reported to us that no—one had heard that particular patient's voice since their admittance to hospital and this very often happens with deeply depressed mentally ill patients. Music has charms indeed to "soothe the savage breast" but an important factor also is that it can be a motivating force for people who are lacking in volition.

Elderly People

There is an increasing need for concerts for very elderly residents in hospital wards.

The benefit that live concerts can bring to elderly people is, as one hospital said recently, "immeasurable". The colour, the warmth of the artists' personalities and being able to hear again the music they have known and loved in the past can mean so much. We are keenly aware of the value of music as an aid to reminiscence, often enabling people to recall the past and through this, helping to re—inforce their present sense of identity.

Concerts help to combat a feeling of loneliness and isolation which is experienced by so many who are in long term care, and they are a welcome break from the day–to–day routine. People are reassured that the outside world still cares. There have been many cases where the staff have been amazed at the reaction of those in their care and have told us how much insight they have gained into their patients' background and tastes, again commenting that they do not seem like the same people when they are alert and happy during and after a concert.

Hospices

Hospices require the greatest sensitivity in approach and in presentation. Not all the patients are there to end their days – some may be in for brief periods, for respite care, or for pain control.

Concerts not only give people a chance to hear a live professional performance, but music can be valuable as a catharsis, bringing emotions to a head and frequently helping patients to begin to come to terms with their illness. We are told again and again how the release of tension brought by the music can open the way for the support and counselling which is of such immense value.

There is benefit to families and friends also, providing a fresh topic to talk about with loved ones and creating something memorable which can be shared together. We hear, too, of patients surfacing from a coma during a bedside concert and we have had many special requests to play for a dying patient.

One of our hospices told us:

> "It was arranged for the harpist to sit and play at the patient's bedside. He was apparently comatose but, on hearing the music, opened his eyes and reached out his arms to his wife and daughter. For some moments they were able to kiss, hug and cry while the harpist continued to play. Witnessing this profoundly affected the emotions of the onlookers as well."

We are frequently told that the music has lifted the mood of the whole hospice, cheering the staff after perhaps a day in which they may have lost several patients. I feel it is important to be aware of the pressures on the carers and we must cater, too, for their wellbeing.

Children

Children's wards in the general hospitals are not always the easiest situations in which to work, due to the wide variety of illnesses we may encounter and the difficulty of catering for the wide age range. Some patients may only be a few months old, cared for in the same ward as those in their early teens.

On the acute wards a live performance, of course, provides a most welcome change to the hospital scene, helping everyone to forget for a while their illness and all that it involves. Music is a valuable way of reducing the stress which may build up on a busy ward, producing a more relaxed and happy atmosphere which is greatly appreciated by the parents as well as the staff and children.

Musicians

This chapter would not be complete without a word about some of the problems and also the rewards experienced by artists working in hospitals.

It can be the unpredictability of the different situations which is stressful. Despite careful briefing and thought, musicians can feel that their programme is unsuitable. There may be, as I have already mentioned, an inappropriate response, or no response at all.

At the last moment the hospital may change the venue and also the audience. An artist will have to work perhaps in a corridor, or with the patients all round them, or even out of sight. The room may be unbearably hot and stuffy, and it is not always possible to ask patients to refrain from smoking. This can be a special problem for singers and wind players, but it has to be faced without comment as a smoking ban would mean that many patients would not wish to attend the concert.

There is no warm-up period in a hospital concert and the attention must be held from the very first moment. Our experience has shown us that to be successful in this work musicians should be able to move round among the patients, holding their hands, kneeling by a wheelchair, responding to requests, while using all the communication skills of touch, eye contact and voice.

An important part of any concert is the visual aspect. Many of our artists change their costume several times and this is enormously appreciated, even by people with visual disabilities who love to feel the different textures.

Patients welcome the chance to see instruments close up, to run their fingers over the strings of the harp or to feel the movement of an accordian.   All this helps to provide a central point for the attention, and enables patients to be actively involved in the performance through listening and participating.   In all hospital concerts the utmost flexibility is required.   It is the needs of the patients which must be paramount.

For pianists – some pianos are reasonably adequate, but many cannot be brought up to pitch and you could find two octaves missing; the piano might collapse in your lap; you might discover it is used as the hospital ashtray, has been eaten by moths or a mouse might run out!   (These are all things which have happened to our artists.)   The hospitals do their best but, due to the heat on the wards and lack of funds for tuning, a properly maintained piano is a luxury.   An electric piano/keyboard is invaluable.

The amount of benefit the patients can derive from a concert corresponds directly to the ability of the musicians to build a relationship with their audience, to communicate with the most frail, withdrawn or apathetic individuals and to create an informal atmosphere in which the patients can yet enjoy a professional performance, which then becomes a shared experience between the artists and their listeners.

To catch the imagination and hold the attention of a hospital audience is an enormous challenge and a unique chance to use our gifts where they are most needed.

"These concerts provide a chance to give back something to the profession that I love so dearly". (Nigel Perona-Wright of "Dragonsfire")

Every day that passes I am more than ever convinced that music is unsurpassed as a means of communication.   Being non-verbal and non-threatening, it nevertheless, as Plato says; "has the power to penetrate the inmost recesses of the human soul.

It is my conviction that the healing power of music for a hospital audience is indeed "unlimited"."

* *

From June Cooper, Cranage Hall Hospital, Visual Handicap Unit, Crewe

"I am writing to thank you for a most excellent concert. We had a most positive response from all our residents. I was a bit dubious regarding the venture because it was a string quartet, but you could have heard a pin drop! The residents were spellbound by the music and the staff enjoyed it too and found it a very refreshing experience. The Kreutzer Quartet were excellent and formed a good rapport with the audience, during and after the concert.

I have been asked by the residents if they could have more concerts like this. Once again – thank you.

From Sister Aine Cox, Matron, St. John's Hospice, Lancaster

"Concerts are of great value to patients, staff, and indeed to the performers.

To patients – they bring people from 'outside' into the Hospice. The performers are young, they usually dress up and they help to revive memories and enable patients to forget their worries and illness for a short period. The performance is like a gesture of love and remembrance from the community and the youth (the people of tomorrow!) and is an indication that they are still of value and have not been forgotten.

They are good for the staff too – they give them something to talk about with the patients.

I feel they are a challenge to the young performers. It is a completely new kind of audience, quite different from a commercial one. It can be a 'shifting' audience as their concentration span is poor and they may not be able to sit for long. Memories – painful or emotional may be raised, giving rise to tears.

The music requested may not be of the kind the musicians would choose, but their aim is to give pleasure. The musician will not always get the response or applause he might expect from the usual Concert audience so he has to perform for the joy of performing and out of a sincere wish to bring pleasure to this special group of people.

The rewards can be very great."

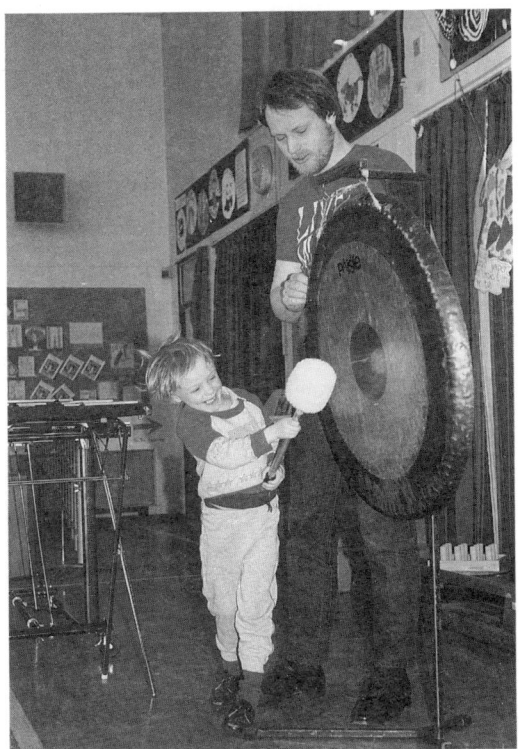

Figure 1: Andrew Whettham. "Percussion Calls the Tune".
Longsight Park School, Manchester.

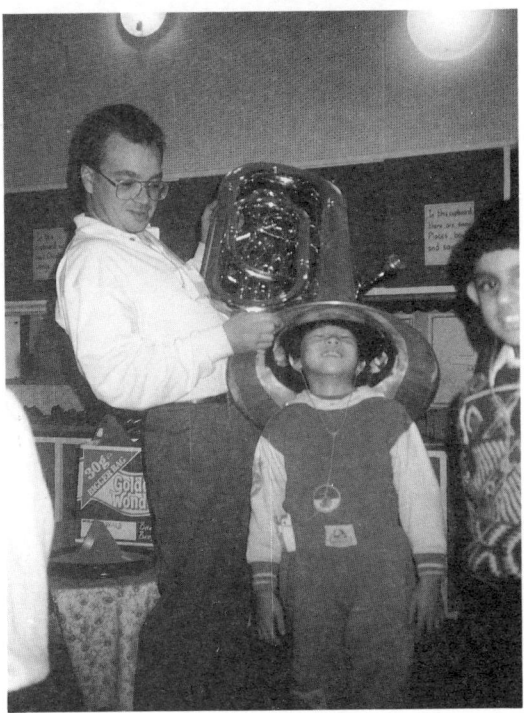

Figure 2: Gavin Woods. Phoenix Brass Quintet. Park Dean School, Oldham.

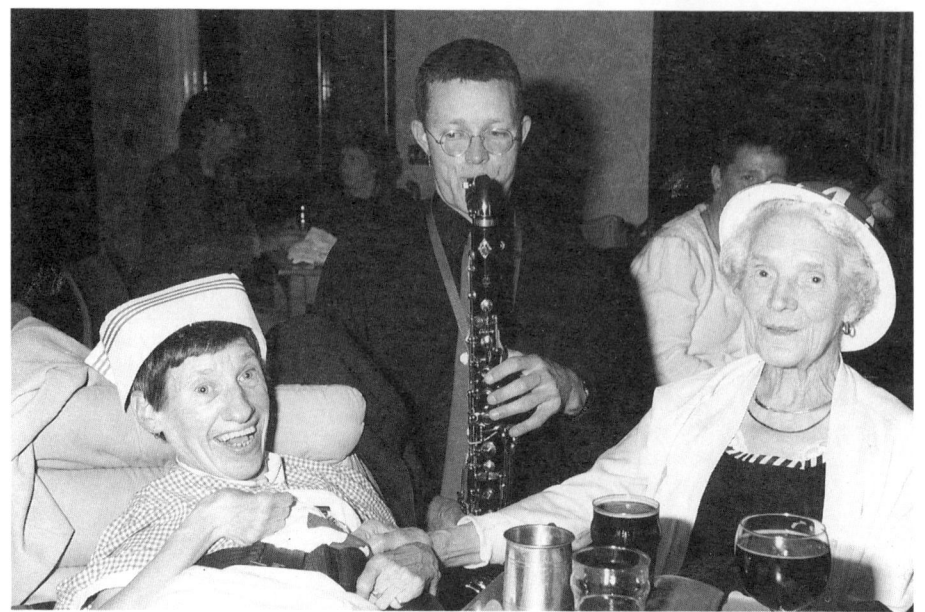

Figure 3: Nick Hayes. No Strings Attached. Jubilee Centre, Bolton.
Photo: Steve Yates.

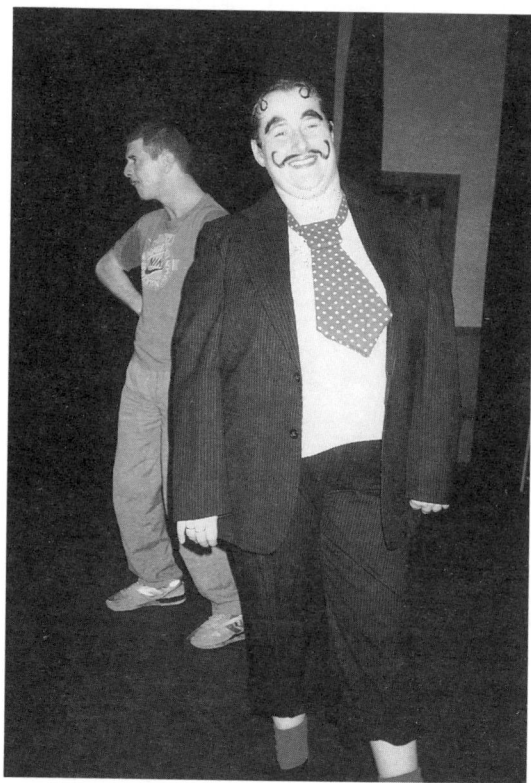

Figure 4: 2 members of the cast of "A Horse Designed by a Committee".
Jubilee Centre, Bolton.

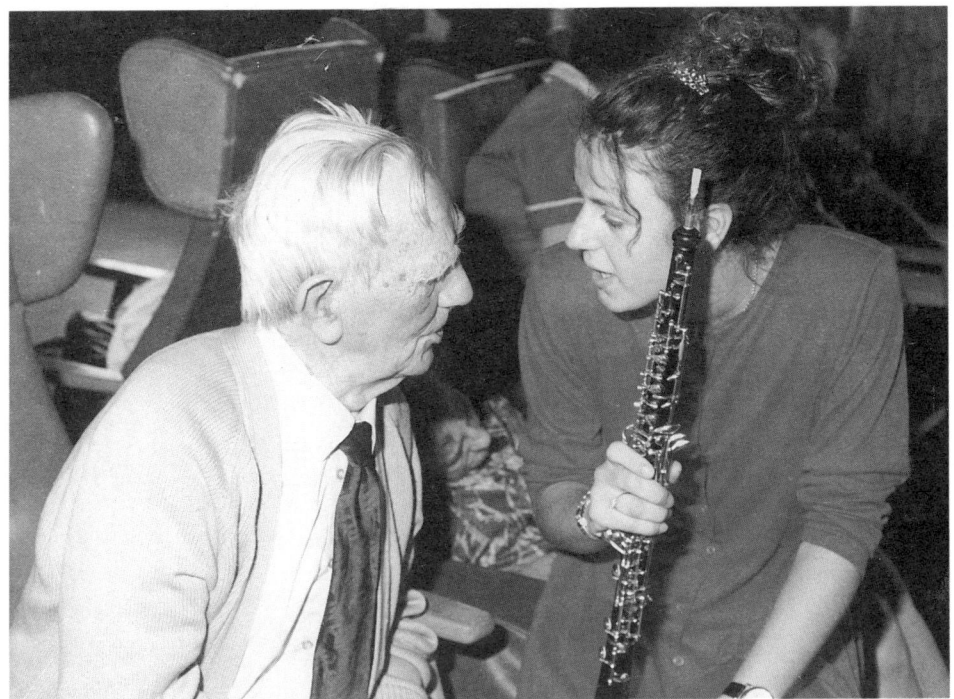

Figure 5: Rachael Clegg. Chione Oboe Trio. Manchester Royal Infirmary.
Photo: Steve Yates.

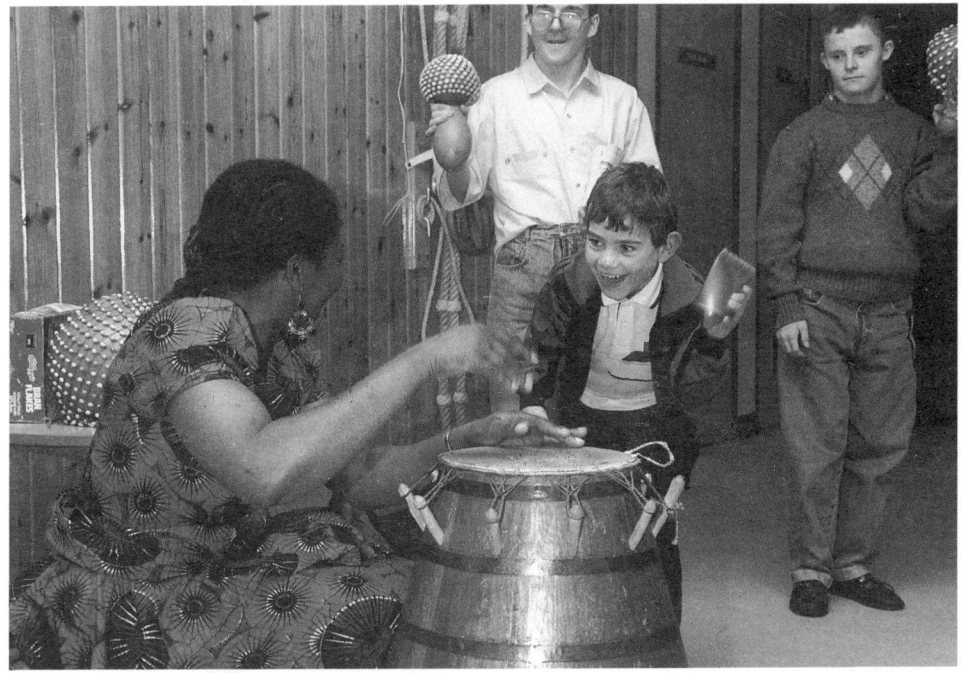

Figure 6: Miso'shi. Helland School, Manchester.
Photo: Steve Yates.

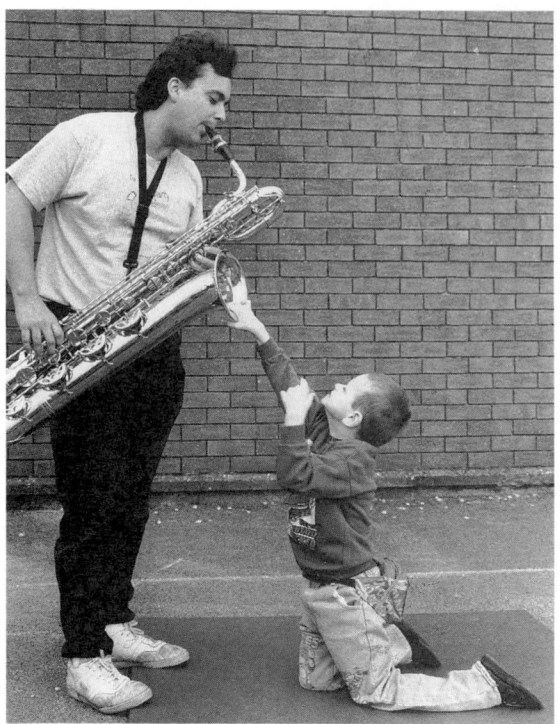

Figure 7: Jon Rebbeck. Apollo Saxophone Quartet. Valley School, Stockport.
Photo: Mark Little.

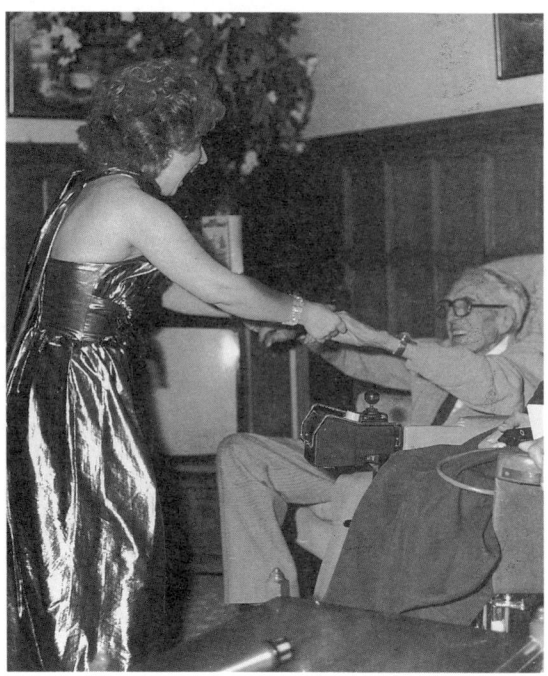

Figure 8: Kay Carman (Soprano). Knowle Park Nursing Home, Cranleigh.
Photo: Peter N. Felton.

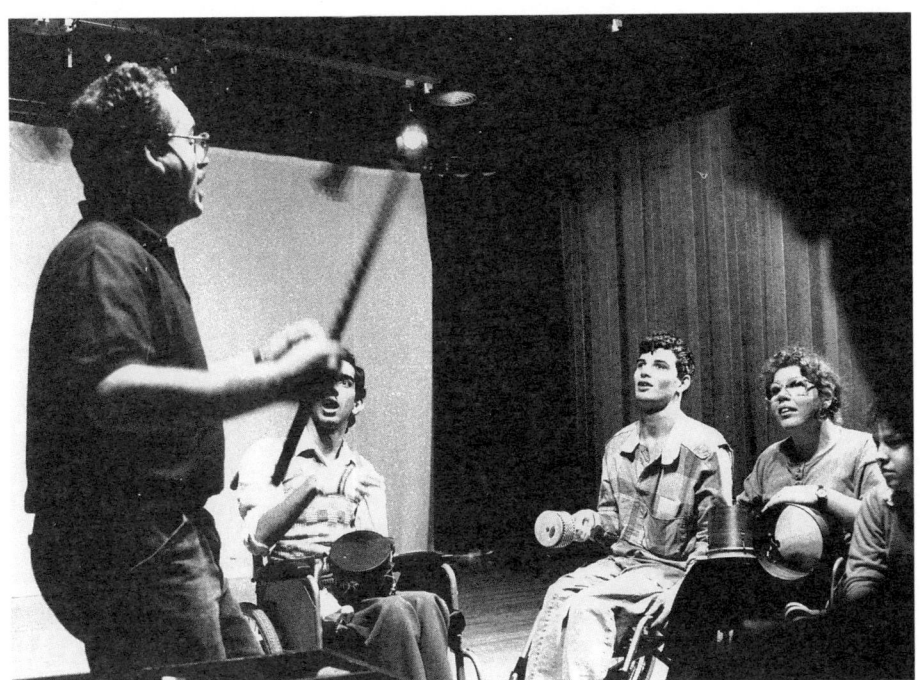

Figure 9: Kenton Mann with students at Beaumont College, Lancaster.
Photo: Mary Jones.

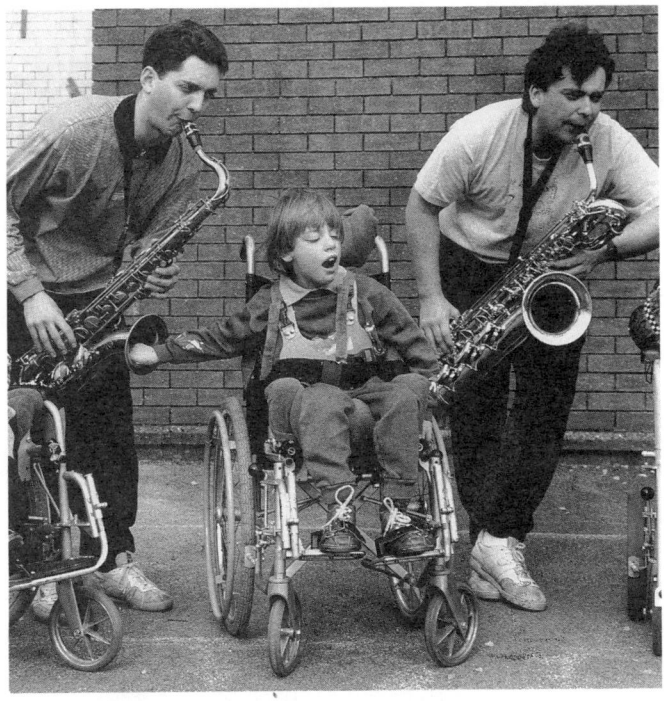

Figure 10: Andy Scott and Jon Rebbeck of Apollo Saxophone Quartet.
Valley School, Stockport.
Photo: Mark Little.

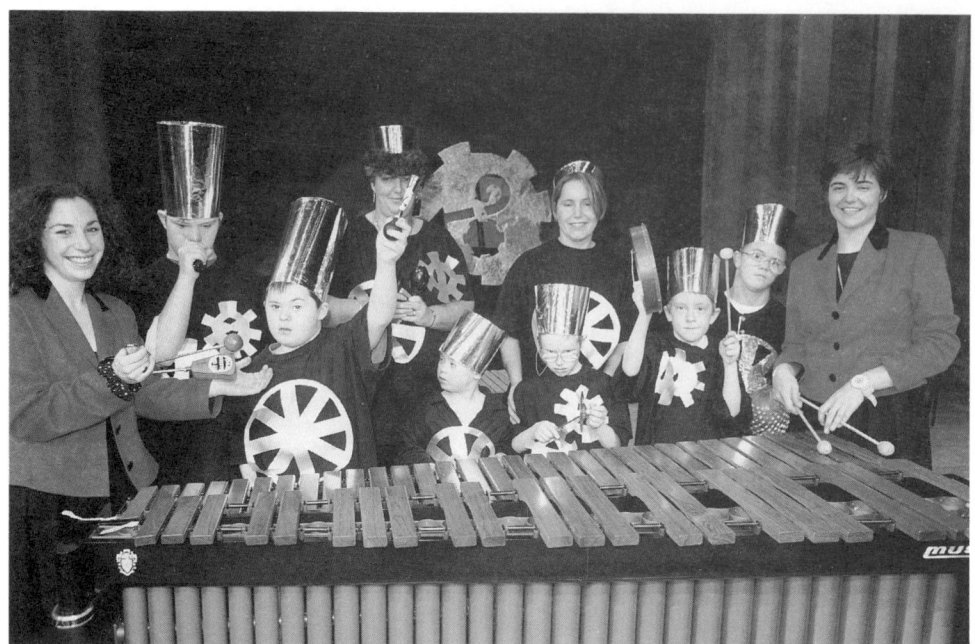

Figure 11: Patricia Allardyce and Sarah Wood. Off the Beaten Track.
Leecroft School, Manchester.
Photo: Manchester Evening News.

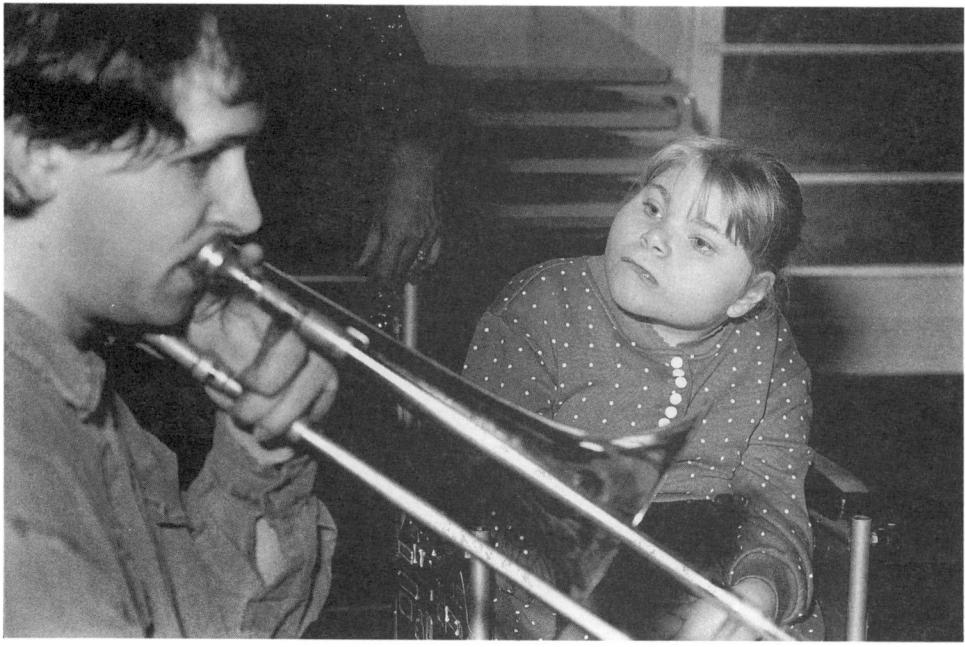

Figure 12: David Chambers. Phoenix Brass Quintet. Tor View School, Haslingden.
Photo: Nigel Hillier.

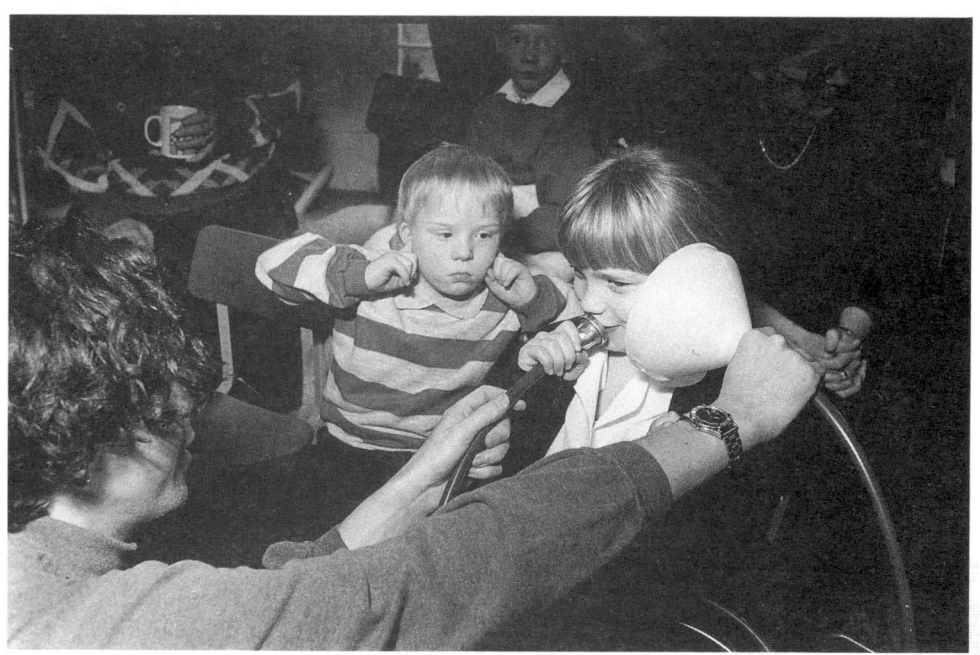

Figure 13: Jason Glover. Bone Idols. Tor View School, Haslingden.
Photo: Nigel Hillier.

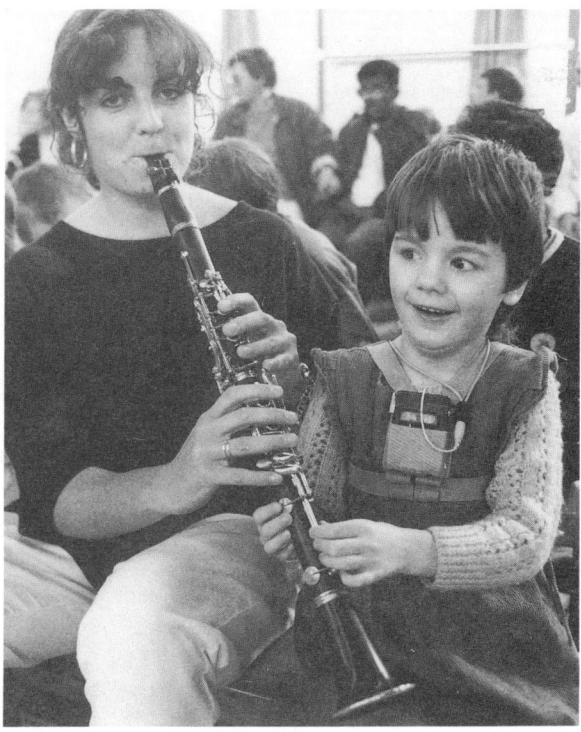

Figure 14: Gina with clarinettist friend from No Strings Attached.
Schools for the Deaf.

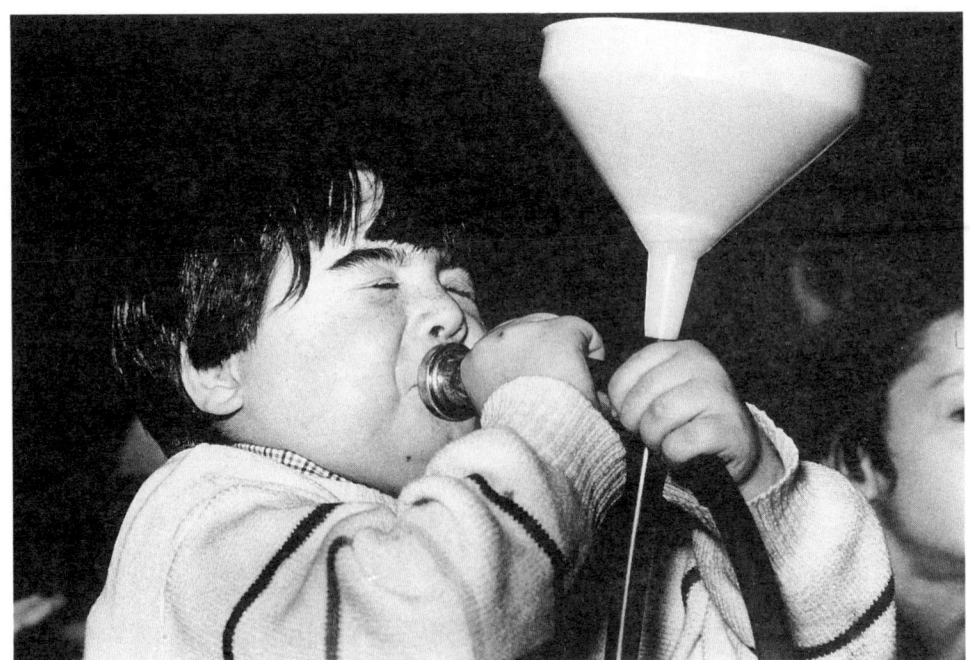

Figure 15
Photo: Nigel Hillier

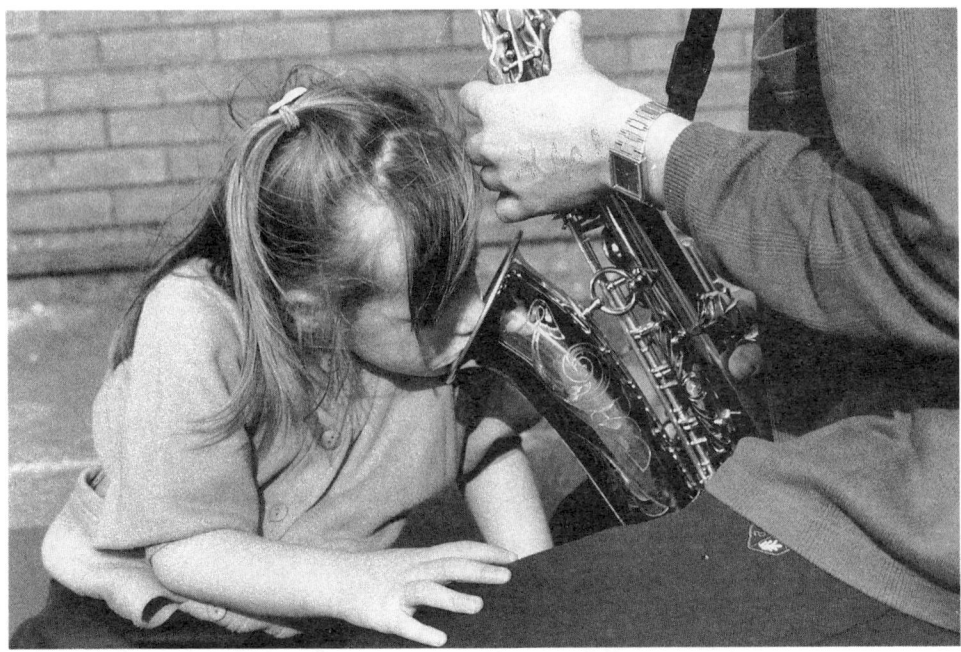

Figure 16: Valley School, Stockport.
Photo: Mark Little.

Residents in Elderly Persons' Homes

"Music, the greatest good that mortals know,
And all of heaven we have here below." (Joseph Addison)

It is a sad fact that modern Western societies do not value their elderly people. The confused, forgetful and "unattractive" have no system through which they can contribute. Without community support, families can not cope with relatives who are demanding yet dependent. It is these people who become resident in Elderly Person's Homes.

The home, funded privately or by Social Services, should provide a safe, warm environment and a balanced diet for its residents. Caring for the body, however, does not stimulate the mind. Institutional life, coupled with the insularity of the home, can lead to mental stagnation. There is a growing recognition that stimulating the mind leads to improved physical health in the elderly and that Art, including live music, is an effective means to this end.

As the home functions on a 24 hour, 365 days a year basis, the staff work in shifts. There will probably be an Officer in Charge, a Deputy, a Third Officer and a team of care staff runnning the home. It is possible that, after your initial phone call, preliminary visit and performance you will have seen a different Senior Officer each time. A written list of details (chairs, start time, arrival times etc) is a good idea. Leave one in the office on your pre-concert visit.

Although your visits will be arranged with senior staff, you will actually be working with care staff during your performance. Care staff may well be part-time and not fully briefed on what to expect. Just getting the residents organised will require the co-operation of the care staff, so take time to gain their good will. A shared joke, small talk or just a smile can change the atmosphere completely.

Your Audience

Elderly people are not stupid – they are just old. For a variety of reasons (institution life, mental or physical illness) some may have lost social skills which most of us take for granted, leading to unpredictable behaviour. It is quite possible that a member of your audience may call out while you are playing, get up and leave the room or strike up a conversation with a neighbour in the middle of a soft passage. Don't let this put you off.

Remember that, for this audience, the atmosphere you get is the one you create. More than in any other venue, it is crucial to find time to talk to the residents as individuals. These are people whom society has put "on the shelf" and they may well have ceased to regard themselves, their opinions and reactions as valuable. By taking the trouble to put together an accessible programme and performing for the residents, you are saying that their value for *you* is undiminished.

Touch, as a means of communication, is terribly important and the simple act of shaking hands with everyone will ensure their attention to your playing. Make time to have a cup of tea with residents before, after or even during the concert.

The Performance

Your performance space is unlikely to be "user friendly". Elderly people cannot tolerate cold and draughts, so the room will probably be stuffily warm. It may well be carpeted, full of furniture and have a low ceiling – all of which add up to a dead acoustic. Certainly for wind players these are strength sapping conditions, so be prepared.

The first thing you will feel is the lack of audience "buzz". This does not mean that there is a lack of interest – just a lack of energy. The residents may be frail and unable to give a round of applause or call out answers to questions. This doesn't mean that they don't want to, or that they are unappreciative – you have to assume the interest and keep performing and projecting.

* *

From Ann Morisy, London Diocesan Board for Social Responsibility

The Measure of our Days

Putting work with frail elderly people into a wider context.

The booking which entails a performance in a residential home for the elderly may well bring a host of mixed emotions. It is worthwhile unravelling the reasons for such ambivalence, not least because the blossoming of the number of elderly people, especially those over 80, is just beginning. Demographers estimate that numbers will increase until around 2030 when those who were born during the post–war baby boom will reach old age.

Work with the frail elderly is therefore a major growth area, and it will be so for the time it takes for today's young musicians to themselves become old.   And it is here that lies the rub, unlike many other engagements in the community, when confronted by the frailness of those in a residential or nursing home, we are also confronted by the fact that we are all caught up in the same process. Those who sit in armchairs arranged around the perimeter of the lounge at the Laurels Rest Home represent what we fear we may become.   Tim Booth, himself the proprietor of a residential home, commented in an address he entitled "Home Truths":

> "Looking at today's residents people ask to be spared the same fate, saying that they hope they don't come to that.   This is not just a fear of growing old.   It is, above all, a dread of what they see as the purposelessness and powerlessness of residential life and its empty hours".

For all of us there is a temptation to deny our basic solidarity in this most human of processes.   Howard Becker highlights our capacity to repress the inevitability of our own death, and thus when we sit alongside the frail elderly we are brought uncomfortably close to having to acknowledge our own creatureliness and finitude, profoundly threatening the narcissism, or self love, which we cultivate. According to Becker, we are caught-up in a "terrifying dilemma", since:

> "Man is literally split in two: he has an awareness of his splendid uniqueness in that he sticks out of nature with a towering majesty, and yet he goes back into the ground a few feet in order to blindly and dumbly rot and disappear for ever." (Becker, 1973)

For the musician who, for the very best professional reasons, has built up a degree of self-esteem and self confidence, it is a rude confrontation, and understandably the insults of ageing may be such that the performance in the residential home is filled with a deep seated dread.

Some sociological reasons can be added to this psychological reason as to why performance in a residential home can be arduous. The undeniable fact is that the elderly are culturally despised, and perhaps this is not unrelated to the fact that the frail elderly are predominantly female.   In a society where the dead have no mythical power over the living there is nothing to counteract this serious undervaluing of the humanity and dignity of the old.   Curtin writes:

"I have learned that a culture which equates material possessions with success, and views the frantic, compulsive consumer as the perfect citizen can afford little space for the aged human being. They are past competing, they are out of the game. We live in a culture which endorses human obsolescence ... to the junk heap, the nursing home, the retirement village, the 'Last Resort'." (Curtin, 1972)

Each time the professional musician accepts a gig in a residential home, he or she is not just in the business of entertainment they are also in the business of 'counter–culture'. In giving of their best to those who are culturally despised the musician is working against the unstated, but nonetheless real, undervaluing of the aged women who sit passively in the upholstered armchairs in the lounge.

Alongside these rather scholarly factors which work against involvement with the aged human being, there is also a very basic, practical reason which may underlie hesitancy in relation to work with the frail elderly. That is the lurking doubt as to whether the musician's contribution makes any difference, or even whether it is noticed, let alone whether it is remembered or of benefit.

For those who sit passively in the lounge of a residential home, not only are they locked into the deadening routine of institutional living, day in, day out. This deadening experience comes on top of possibly many years living alone, with a diminishing number of meaningful contacts. Professor Rabbit of Manchester University talks of boredom as being as great a threat to life as cigarette smoking. In the light of this it might be expected that the atmosphere for the concert or performance relies almost completely upon the performers and response has to be prompted and participation coaxed.

Until recently, it has been assumed that with ageing a fairly rapid decline takes place in both cognitive and intellectual ability. However, researchers now propose a 'plasticity model' to describe the relationship between ageing and cognitive capacity. Essentially, this model emphasises that if a decline occurs in cognitive capacity then it is likely that it can be reversed through appropriate stimulating, thus for elderly people a stimulating environment is vital.

Moss and Halamandaris in their book "Too Old, Too Sick, Too Bad" refer to work in an American nursing home in which two thirds of the 67 elderly patients were classified as 'heavycare', meaning that they needed help with dressing, washing, toileting and feeding. As a result of restorative activities, 1 year later only 9 were classified as 'heavycare'. The restorative activity was a weekly poetry appreciation class. In order to understand how such a near miraculous transformation can be brought about it is necessary to unravel the dynamics which are set in motion by something like an art class or music workshop which involves those who are elderly and frail.

For example, attendance, and preferably participation, in a regular event or workshop enables a group of elders to share the same activity, and this shared experience generates conversation between the participants. The staff have something 'good' to express interest in, and further conversation is generated. Thus there is new material for remembering and for relating to other residents, staff, and to family and friends when they visit.

An underestimated dynamic is the restoration of the motivation to please or impress someone of significance. By being in the company of the tutor, or adept musician, the desire to please is rekindled, so more trouble is taken over appearance and mobility is enhanced because of the sense of eagerness. Along with this the habit of attending to the environment, the people, the objects in it, is re-awakened, so that memory improves or at least is not lost.

The research undertaken by Moss and Halamandaris – and similar research by Sylvia Poulden, Jean Mulford and Ruth Michaels to mention just a few – refers to the regaining of continence, and they describe how this comes about:

> "Greater attention to the world, to herself, to time and place, to other people and to their responses, is instrumental in restoring an awareness of internal stimuli, of taking heed, of looking ahead. Thus a greater initiative, a responsibility for the self, a recognition of other's opinions about oneself and a restoration of self-respect may well lead to the growth of continent behaviour. Apathy has been overcome." (Moss and Halamandaris, 1977)

It would be naive to think that the occasional concert could achieve such a profound change and restoration of faculties. However, a regular hour long workshop over a period of three months would begin to have an appreciable effect. If considered solely in terms of cost effectiveness, the contribution of the musician to the demands made by those in need of heavy care, would bring a significant saving in other staff costs. Moreover, the contribution the musician makes to the humanising of a total institution such as a residential or nursing home is inestimable.

In many ways music is more conducive to the stimulation of those who have become deeply passive than is poetry or story reading. In listening to a musician, initially, demands are made only on the most passive senses, those of watching and listening. The distinctiveness of a performance is that it has the capacity to call forth appropriate behaviour from those who are otherwise confused. Furthermore, the presence of a clearly professional musician flatters, and it is well known that flattery illicits in people (of all ages) the desire to please and to give of their best.

The presence, in a residential home or day centre for the elderly, of those who normally perform for a large audience, and possibly for a large fee, speaks of esteem rather than the disdain which the frail elderly often experience. Thus the professional musician, in drawing alongside 'the decrepit old woman', engages in radical 'counter–cultural' activity. When that drawing alongside takes place on a regular basis clear messages are transmitted to a range of people: To the elderly person – You matter to me; To her relatives – Your mother is someone I value; To the care staff – The environment in which you work as a care assistant is one which is significant to me. The potency of such messages is enhanced by the fact that they are carried by someone who is not a part of the recognised 'caring professions', who tend to carry such affirming messages in a manner which is calculated to 'do–good'.

Patrick White, in his classic work "Riders in the Chariot" writes thus of his unbecoming, post–menopausal heroine and of those who could see beyond her appearance and lowly social standing:

"From behind her great beam, under the stretchy cardigan, she might have appeared something of a joke, except for the few who happened to perceive that she also wore the crown." (White, 1961)

With all the associated pathos, it is this capacity to perceive the crown which is worn by those who are decrepit through having lived a life, which is surely at the heart of an effective engagement with and for frail elderly people.

References

Becker, H. (1973) *The Denial of Death*; New York: The Free Press, p.26.

Curtin, S. R. (1972) *Nobody Ever Died of Old Age*; Boston and Toronto: Little and Brown, pp.195–6.

References to these researchers (Sylvia Poulden, Jean Mulford and Ruth Michaels) and their findings are to be found in Johnson, S. and Philipson, C. (Eds.) *Older Learners: The Challenge of Adult Education*; London: Age Concern/NCVO.

Moss, F.E. and Halamandaris, V.J. (1977) *Too Old, Too Sick, Too Bad*: Nursing Homes in America; Maryland: Aspen Systems Corporation.

White, P. (1961) *Riders in the Chariot*; London: Penguin Modern Classics p.491.

From Pat Hyde, Parklands, Poynton

"I really don't know where to start to say thank you for the concert here last Tuesday.   To start with everything seemed to be so beautifully organised.   The girls came to visit before the concert and had immediate empathy with the residents, and as for the concert, everyone, the residents, the staff, the CSL Director, Mr. Peter Nash, the team leader and myself, thoroughly enjoyed it.   The residents kept saying to me how they'd enjoyed themselves, they didn't realise such music was possible on those kind of instruments*.   What a change to have a live performance, how much they'd enjoyed watching the girls enjoying themselves, what charming girls they were.   Would they come again?   I don't think I've ever organised such a successful evening and given so many people pleasure.   Especially as there had been one or two noses turned up at the mere hint of classical music.

Gladys, the resident who adores music (rather than sing songs with guitars and keyboards which we usually have) was in her element, the more so because she loves to see young people perform.

Sarah and Patricia gave of their best but even more important managed to project their love of music and play as though they wanted us to share their love and exuberance.

Thank you again for a most memorable and enjoyable evening."

*   (This performance was given by the percussion duo —
Off The Beaten Track).

Inmates in Prisons

"The excellency of art is in its intensity, capable of making all disagreeables evaporate, from their being in close relationship with beauty and truth." (John Keats)

Anyone applying to visit a prison will be automatically vetted by the Home Office using existing records. This is not as intrusive as it may sound at first. Credit companies and many prospective employers may do exactly the same.

Once cleared for admittance, everything depends on the goodwill of the prison officers. You cannot access your performance space, nor can your audience arrive, without them. If a certain officer does not see the value of your visit there is little you can do about it. It will help, however, if everyone in your group knows the name of the person who booked you and what position, or rank, he holds. All uniformed services are hierarchyic and have their own terms of address. Recognition of this will help as you negotiate your way around the establishment.

"Am I at risk?" No. You and your instrument are probably more at risk getting into an orchestral pit than you are in a prison.

Women may feel very uncomfortable at the prospect of going into a male prison but there is really no need to worry. It might be the case that there will be 'risque' heckling from individuals but it could just as easily be aimed at the men in your group!

The Performance

Your audience will be glad to see you and, like every other audience, the mood may change a good deal from piece to piece. Loud criticism and comments on your music or introductions are not uncommon and are usually a sign of interest rather than derision.

Remand prisoners constitute a transient prison population and this often leads to less provision for outside stimuli. They may have been waiting months for their trial – possibly in several prisons. It is not difficult to imagine the frustration that this can cause.

You must not expect an ideal performance area. You may be asked to play in a classroom or on a wing but, more than likely, you will be playing in the Chapel – usually the most pleasant room in the building – so this is a bonus.

The following section by Sara Lee shows what can be achieved through long–term project work with inmates allowing time to build mutual trust and respect.

* *

From Sara Lee, "No Strings Attached" (A Quartet of Clarinets), Music Tutor, HMP Wormwood Scrubs

The overiding factor that is always mentioned by people who come into the prison to work is the abundance of enthusiasm the men have. This has always been my experience, not just as regards music but any live activity.

Getting any sort of performance to any community venue is important, especially so to a prison, which can be so sterile. The men have limited access to music – radios and a few tapes are virtually the sole providers – so the value of a live performance is unquestionable. Obviously the ideal would be to have a pre–concert visit but in the prison situation this can be impractical, which means that groups have to come in and perform 'cold' so to speak.

As with any venue, aural and visual stimulation are important – the audience will be interested in the dress, the introductions and the instruments as well as the music. After a recent concert and asking how much the instruments cost, one of the audience said "that clarinet's worth over £1000 you say? I'm gutted! A mate once asked me to flog one quickly for him and I reckoned I'd done well to get £100!"

The audience will be as mixed as in a concert hall, bar the fact they will be either all men or all women. As a result the programme choice can be really varied. The appreciation is often immediate and audible: regarding Duke Ellington's *Don't get around much any more* ... "Well I certainly don't mate!" and (performer to audience) "We'd love a chat afterwards if you've got time"... "I've got fifteen years, is that enough?" Standing ovations are normal and are *always* genuine.

As important as the concert is the tea and chat afterwards. The staff always remain in the background allowing the audience time to get into conversation with the performers. This time is *never* long enough – so many questions have to be asked of each other and the call for the end always seems to come at the crucial moment!

The clarinet quartet 'No Strings Attached' perform regularly in HMP Wormwood Scrubs and we learned at the outset never to underestimate the simplest things – many of the men have commented on the way we move when we play, how they've noticed the eye contact we have and also the confusion when one of us thinks another one is going to introduce a piece so neither of us do – then two of us try to – all things that we barely think of during a performance as it's second nature to us, but all things that are very interesting to a group of people whose contact with every day occurences is so limited.

We've found it a great place to try out new pieces and programmes. As well as an appreciative audience, you get an honest appraisal of the music and the performance and also many extra ideas of what to say in introductions that will be of interest to any audience.

"I was apprehensive before my first visit but immediately found it a very positive situation for music which doesn't really exist anywhere else. Most of the men would probably never have been to this kind of concert outside but they were very open–minded and interested in everything we did and said." (Andrew Sparling, No Strings Attached)

I was first introduced to music in prisons in 1984 as part of a newly formed course at the Guildhall School of Music and Drama. The object of the course was to introduce music and performers to new audiences and surroundings, and one of our first term projects was to visit HMP Wormwood Scrubs and give a concert to a group of inmates from the long term wing. Unusually for the course there was no prior visit to the prison – we had been used to visiting venues beforehand to meet the people who would be attending the concert and to discuss programme ideas, but due to the high security of Wormwood Scrubs we were left to plan a programme based on instinct.

The concert was to start at 6.00 p.m. but we were to arrive before 5.30 p.m. to enable security checks to be carried out. This took all of the half hour allotted and the men began to arrive as we were setting up. Our programme was immediately rearranged to incorporate a piece written by one of the inmates, a piece for oboe and cello which we spontaneously transcribed for two clarinets and cello. Frank had brought the piece over on the off–chance he could hear how it sounded – the first public performance of his piece and in fact the first time he had heard any of his music played.

The whole concert was a huge success, extremely moving for the performers and thrilling for the audience. During a discussion with staff at the end of the concert, the Education Officer realised the potential music could have within the prison and asked whether any of the group would be interested in working within the prison on a regular basis.

For a long while I ran a practical music class for one session a week. Ten men brought their instruments and we wrote songs, taught each other many things, and went away refreshed. I quickly realised that the guitar was by far the most popular instrument. Being a clarinettist, I had to enlist the help of the men who were sufficiently proficient guitarists to help the beginners so that I could concentrate on explaining how to *write* music and furthermore how to understand what you'd written – also how to rehearse and get a performance together. As time has gone on, these last two factors, rehearsal and performance – have become very important parts of our sessions together.

(At this point I have to add that the logistics of organising in a prison can be traumatic – the simplest thing like walking a group of ten men from 'a' to 'b' can be a problem if there are no officers available for escorting – we've just always been fortunate to have governors and officers who are eager for new things to happen and who will volunteer their services to ensure the smooth running of a project.)

It was quickly becoming apparent that there was a great deal of untapped talent within the prison and if I was going to get the most out of our time together then somehow I had to arrange a time and place for a performance. The place was not a problem – we decided to use the prison chapel for an evening. This quickly escalated to three evenings, as the men wanted to experience something other than a one-off.

Several performers were involved in a mixture of music, poetry and improvisation and this was backed up with an exhibition of artwork produced mainly by the full-time art group. Our audiences consisted of one night for invited members of the public and one night for the rest of D wing, and the reception was tremendous. The performers, none of whom had worked in front of an audience before, and the majority of whom had not played/written music/poetry before the start of their sentence, were planning the next project even before this one had finished! My class grew steadily as the men realised that you didn't necessarily have to know or play anything before you joined and it was with an enlarged group that the London Sinfonietta came in to work.

The London Sinfonietta have an excellent education programme and fortunately for us have continued and developed their working relationship with Wormwood Scrubs. Long as well as short term projects are of immense value within the prison system. The Sinfonietta's projects, as well as being of unquestionable musical value, have also been valuable as a source of human contact, both professional and personal.

> "I've found that performance restores in a person that sense of responsibility, self–discipline and individuality which we as prisoners tend to lack. Interaction is essential, as is strong rapport with fellow performers. Again, these are social skills which prison life can erode." (Matthew)

Undoubtedly the more you put into the job the more you get out and it's certainly advisable to try anything you feel brave enough to have a go at. An example would be our most recent venture, putting on a week's run of the musical 'Oliver'. We only had three months of rehearsal during which we had to overcome hurdles such as men with lead roles being transferred to other prisons three weeks before performances, vital rehearsals cancelled due to lack of officer cover – all potentially awkward situations. But the men know how the system can work sometimes, and were ready, very willing and able to swap parts at the last moment and to organise rehearsals in their cells to make sure no time was lost. It is often necessary to look to the staff and men for support and advice – they know the system better than anyone and can help you work within it.

Prisons are a much written about (though little known) area of society which I personally have found extremely rewarding to work in – just another community group who find themselves in more unusual surroundings. It was a completely unknown quantity years ago. I feel glad that I went into prison with an open mind. This allowed me to form my own opinions based on fact rather than fiction. The few preconceptions that I did have were soon dispersed.

I have found an enthusiasm and commitment to the work which is rare outside. True, the men find themselves with more time than most to practice but time is still valuable to them and they structure their lives accordingly. For whatever reason, they find themselves doing anything up to 20 years and if they can find an outlet for their creativity through music, then we work together. I have often been asked 'how will music possibly be of worth when the man is released?" Whether or not the individual pursues music as a career upon release doesn't matter. The discipline required learning any skill can be used and applied to so many other fields of life, not just in the one it began in.

"I've only been playing the clarinet a year and I was scared, wondering if I could do it.   Mainly because my counting was weak, but after five rehearsals, listening to the quality of the players around me gave me a firm idea of how to go about things."   (Michael − joining No Strings Attached for the performance of *Oliver*)

"Working within your own capabilities and then expanding them and watching fellow inmates do likewise is very exciting.   When the combined effort of everyone involved finally culminates in a successful performance, the personal and joint sense of achievement is a "high" I've never before experienced.   And that's something coming from a lifer." (Matthew)

Christmas card, 1991

"To Sara, the one who helped me find my brains, Yeah!"

Audience Involvement

"Music is essentially useless, as life is: but both lend utility to their conditions." (George Santayana)

If you have made a pre-concert visit to the venue, and based your programme upon information obtained, you have already gone a long way towards involving the audience in your music. The more that you get your audience actively involved in your performance, the more they will enjoy it, and the more you will *all* get out of it.

Audience involvement will enhance listening skills, underline musical effects, draw attention to instrumental techniques, encourage criticism, comments and feedback and – by all these means further the audience's enjoyment.

Aim for involvement in almost every piece that you play. This sounds like a tall order, so here are some ideas:–

For Children

(Some of these suggestions can be adapted for adult audiences).

As you introduce your instruments, demonstrate the range of each and ask the children to raise their hands as the notes go higher – and lower them as you play down the range. When you can see that most children are responding, turn this into a game and play high and low notes alternately, slowly at first – then faster.

Pick two short contrasting pieces – one fast and one slow. Talk about speed and encourage children to beat time – small movements with just their fingers for the quick piece and large arm movements for the slow one.

Recognition of loud and soft can be shown by spreading arms wide for loud (mind your neighbour) and closing hands together tight for soft passages. Stand up when the music gets louder and sit down slowly as it gets softer. Pick the right music for all these activities. Concentrate on one musical effect at a time – and then its opposite.

Your own involvement is important. In all these games, encourage and applaud responses. Extravagant praise will ensure attention and a quick response to the next game.

When you ask questions of an audience of children, always say "put up your hand if you can tell me ......". This avoids the unintelligible burst of sound you will get if you ask the question of everyone. "Not quite" or "nearly" are encouraging responses to the wrong answers. Repeat the right answer clearly yourself so that everyone has heard it.

One of your pieces could be designed to benefit from a simple percussion accompaniment. By now you have noticed several children with a very good sense of rhythm. Ask one or two to come and help you play the next piece. If some children are the "stars" with you, all the others are empathising and therefore listening very hard. Treat your volunteers as part of your group and make sure they know what they are doing. Naturally they get a special round of applause – at the beginning for offering to help and at the end for playing so well. If this (or any part of your programme) works particularly well, play it again with some variation – different volunteers, instruments, rhythmic accompaniment, dynamic etc.

(The best percussion instruments to use are those which can be held in one hand and hit with the other. Don't use anything wobbly (like triangles) or anything needing a separate beater. Unbreakable single headed drums, tambourines and shakers are probably the best. Don't rely on the school to produce these. Have your own and make sure they are good quality, and washable.)

Include at least one piece that needs everyone to be very quiet – a lullaby perhaps, or music for a quiet summer's evening/midnight at Christmas/whatever. Describe the scene you think the music is about and encourage everyone to shut their eyes and imagine it while you play. Finish *ppp*, and try for that magic five seconds silence at the end before everyone wakes up and claps.

One way to ensure variety and discussion in your programmes is to take a theme. For instance:- plan a concert round different forms of transport – everything from your own feet to donkey rides, trains, submarines and space flight. A journey round the world gives opportunities for very varied musical styles. A concert depicting the Weather or Seasons could start with the present conditions and go on to lots of "do you remember?" and "what does it feel like when . ?" A performance built on the history of your instruments and the sort of music they have played since they were first invented to the present day, is well worth the trouble that it takes to organise.

Write your own music for these programmes, arrange music that you need, be inventive! You will gradually build up a repertoire of programmes that you can adapt to suit any group.

For Every Audience

Characterize the mood of the piece and show how, by the choice of sounds and the way they are used; this mood is created.

Say how long the piece will take to perform; how many sections it has and what happens in each section.

Say how often a theme occurs. Play the theme by itself several times on different instruments at different pitches, using different dynamics.

Emphasise geographical and/or historical connections. Maybe the piece has a very strong Spanish influence – talk about Spain and have castanets/a tamborine/a picture of a flamenco dancer/a map or whatever is appropriate, with you. If you are playing a gavotte – explain how different was the dancing of 200 years ago. The people who danced in elaborate court costumes (high wigs, enormous skirts) couldn't dance very fast, so a gavotte moves sedately.

Instruments

As part of your demonstration of your instruments, members of the audience can be allowed to touch, hold or even "play" one – to press down a key while you blow, or stop a string while you bow.

Show just what your instrument can do – all the horrible sounds as well as the conventional ones. Show the use of some of these sounds in the next piece. Explain which instrument plays what part, and why. Play some parts of the coming piece on their own – bass line/melody line/a repeated rhythmic pattern/a motif.

Comments, criticism and feedback

Like every other part of your programme, this is a two–way process.

Applause *must* be acknowledged. If you ignore compliments, they will dry up. Tell the audience how much you appreciate their applause/their good listening and why this is important to you.

Allow time for questions and use musical demonstrations in your answers.

Encourage comments – how did this piece make you feel/what did it remind you of, and why? Which was your favourite piece/your favourite instrument, and why?

Ask your audience to hold a discussion after the concert. Ask them to write to you, to send you a picture or a poem.

Leave something of yourselves behind – a contact name, address and phone number/a brochure/a signed photograph, and write to your audience thanking them for their welcome and telling them how much *you* enjoyed playing for *them*.

* *

From Marjorie Dickenson, Oakdale School, Tameside, Summer 1989.

The following extracts from the curriculum at a school for pupils with learning difficulties describe the uses of music as part of the general education programme.

Aims of music in special needs

Music, per se, with any child can be used purely and simply for aesthetic pleasure, but in the case of the profoundly handicapped child it can also be used as a 'calming' influence in tense moments or to invoke excitement and stimulate response in a withdrawn child.

Participation, by means of singing and instrumental work can also create heightened awareness in social response through interaction with others in group activity.

Music can also help in the overall development of the profoundly handicapped child in the following ways:–

1. Increasing auditory awareness through experimental sound using pitch, volume, quality of sound, tempo and rhythm leading to discrimination within the area of sound.

2. As an aid to increasing concentration spans and to more specific 'listening' skills.

3. Increased body awareness when using singing games and rhymes where verbal cues need to be transferred to motor responses.

4. As an aid to movement creating a means of non–verbal communication.

5. "Playing" an instrument even at the most basic level provides physical and tactile benefits besides pleasure and fulfillment. It also involves co-ordination of aural, tactile and usually visual senses.

6. Action songs which require a specific response can be used to improve the child's imitative skills.

7. Greater awareness of speech through rhythmic speaking (e.g., nursery rhymes).

8. An increase in the understanding of sound can also be achieved and the child can be encouraged to understand the differences in sound 'quality' e.g., loud, soft etc.

9. Response to rhythm.

10. Music demands response from all of the senses – tactile, visual and aural. Where a sense is defective or non-existent it can be compensated for, or stimulated by another.

11. Music can provide 'security' for the child through its "emotional language" if he is disturbed or emotionally immature.

12. Greater awareness of intonation and tone of voice.

13. The elements of sound can help in the possible creation of primitive sounds such as non-verbal speech, i.e., babbling.

14. Music can encourage discrimination of types of sound.

(The following section will be of very real value if you intend to develop workshop-based performances.)

In Special Needs, music is used as a means of achieving the following aims:-

1. A means of establishing 'communication'. (Ranging from brief eye-contact to making sounds on an instrument.)

2. Attention and co-operation. In order to establish any form of communication it is essential to gain the child's attention and encourage co-operation.

3. Release of emotions/tension/frustration.

4. Encouragement of hand/eye co-ordination – focusing on an instrument/sound-maker and reaching out to touch/hit etc.

5.   Cause and effect. With music the child is instantly rewarded with sound – he/she learns that his action is producing the sound.

6.   Vocalisation. The most natural form of music is the human voice – turn–taking in musical (vocal) "conversation".

7.   Enjoyment. Sessions must be enjoyable to both the child and the teacher.

Responses to look for:–

(i)   A change in breathing pattern
(ii)   Stilling
(iii)   Change in body posture
(iv)   Eye–contact (however brief)
(v)   Looking, or turning towards the source
(vi)   Change in facial expression
(vii)   Vocalising
(viii)   Reaching out towards the instrument
(ix)   Smiling
(x)   Moving (dancing) in response to music.

Any other responses should be noted.

Give the child time to show a response. The teacher must react at the appropriate level for the child.

Benefits which can be aimed at as a long–term objective:–

(i)   Increased awareness – the child is made aware of sounds around him/her by either producing the sound himself or by hearing sounds produced by others. The child who is hypersensitive to sound will need to have these sounds built up gradually along with visual and tactile knowledge of the 'soundmaker' (desensitization).

(ii)   Improved co–ordination – child can learn different techniques through the experience of producing sounds on an instrument, e.g., hitting, scraping, plucking etc.

(iii)   Concentration – extending the period of time in which the child must attend and co–operate.

(iv)   Vocalisation – child may learn to experiment with his voice.

(v)   Group participation/integration – child can learn to participate in group activity – singing/action rhymes.

(vi)   Interaction with one other person – experience of intimate interaction with another person/turn–taking.

(vii)   Instant results – music has the advantage of being an activity (passive or active) in which there is instant response, e.g., the child hits/touches the instrument and gets an immediate result in the sound produced.

(viii)   Discrimination – likes and dislikes in sound.

Equipment

Un–tuned percussion – whatever sound the child makes will not 'clash' with sounds made by the teacher.
Pentatonic scale – tuned instruments.
Assorted sound–makers – not necessarily musical instruments.

General guidelines

a) Start initial/early sessions in as "distraction–free" area as possible.

b) Have all the instruments on hand so as not to disrupt session.

c) Vary length of session according to the response of the child.

d) Make sure the child is in a safe, comfortable position.

e) Allow time for the child to respond.

f) Always start and finish the session with the same routine – so that the child will learn to predict/anticipate what is going to happen.

g) Tape record the session, if possible. (Responses sometimes occur during a session which are not always acknowledged at the time.)

*   Remember:–

Children in Special Needs:–

–   may not be able to turn their heads/body in both directions.
–   may have hearing impairments which mean that certain pitches cannot be heard clearly.
–   may need increased levels of sound.
–   may be slow to respond – give them time.

Give periods of 'silence' in between periods of 'sound' to allow the child time to become aware of the difference.

> "Music becomes a sphere of experience, a means of inter-communication and a basis for activity in which handicapped children can find freedom, in varying degrees, from the malfunctions which restrict their lives."
> (Nordoff & Robbins)

Getting Started -
Access To Your Audience

First, contact agencies specialising in promoting music in the community. They take care of the funding and administration, which leaves you free to develop your repertoire and presentation techniques. There are two such agencies active in the UK at the time of writing.

Live Music Now! is a national scheme for young musicians. Performers under 27 years of age (30 for singers) may audition. Exceptional performing and communication skills are required. Auditions are held throughout the year at several regional centres. If you are accepted in one region, you are automatically eligible for work in all the others.

The Council for Music in Hospitals holds auditions in the Spring and Autumn each year. Only professional musicians with proven experience are selected to audition. Candidates are expected to perform as if in situ, as directed by the panel. There are no fixed age limits.

Arts Council funding is always prioritised. Your project will have to address specific criteria (cultural, geographical, target groups, training etc.) in order to be considered. Council officers will give advice and send you relevant information.

Promoting Your Own Concerts

Financing your own work outside the concert hall is not easy. You will have to be prepared to seek funding in order to put on performances. Fund raising requires a good deal of organisation and is very time consuming. Plan months, if not years, ahead.

Regional Arts Boards

Arts Officers will know the local scene well. Their advice on local priorities, making bids, those likely to be interested in your ideas, will be crucial.

Local Education Authorities

The introduction of LMS (Local Management of Schools) means that central pots of money are disappearing fast. Nevertheless, some central advisory services still exist. Contact this service as your first step towards work in schools.

Social Services

The policy of "Care in the Community" has put a great strain on Social Services funding. At the same time, it is recognised that the arts have an important role in personal development, and targetted funding does exist.

Training

Music Unlimited is also the title of a training programme run by Isabel Farrell and Kenton Mann.

For more information contact:–

Kenton Mann,
Director, Music Unlimited,
Manchester Metropolitan University,
Grosvenor Building,
All Saints,
Manchester M15 6BR.
Tel.   061–247 3623
Fax.   061–236 0820

Addresses

Arts Council of Great Britain,
(Wendy Harpe, Head of Arts and Disability),
14 Great Peter Street,
London SW1P 3NQ.
Tel.   071–333 0100

Arts For Health is a national advisory centre which advocates the use of all the arts, including music, to complement health care. Contact:–

Peter Senior,
Director, Arts for Health,
Manchester Metropolitan University,
All Saints,
Manchester M15 6BY.
Tel. 061–236 8916

The Council for Music in Hospitals (UK) arranges performances specifically in Hospitals and Hospices. Contact:–

Pam Smith,
Director, The Council for Music in Hospitals,
74 Queen's Road,
Hersham,
Surrey KT12 5LW.
Tel. 0932–252809

The Drake Research Project is involved with the research and production of educational resource materials to enable people with severe disabilities to explore the world of music. Contact:–

Adele Drake, Director,
The Drake Research Project,
3 Ure Lodge,
Ure Bank Terrace,
Ripon, North Yorkshire HG4 1JG.
Tel. 0765–604993

Live Music Now! (UK) aims to provide performances of live music for anyone whose age or disability prevents them from attending concert halls. Contact:–

Virginia Renshaw,
Director, Live Music Now!,
4 Lower Belgrave Street,
London SW1W OLJ.
Tel. 071–730 2205

For information and advice, resource papers and newsletters from the National Music and Disability Arts Information Service, contact:-

Laura Crichton,
Director, National Music and Disability Arts Information Service,
Dartington Hall,
Totnes,
Devon TQ0 6EJ.
Tel. 0803-866701

SHARE Music promotes residential courses in music and theatre with special opportunities and facilities for people with physical disabilities. Contact:-

Dr. Michael Swallow,
15 Deramore Drive,
Belfast BT9 5JQ.
Tel. 0232-669042

The above addresses apply to the UK. Readers in other countries may well find organisations with similar aims via public libraries and other national and local information systems.

Performers' Perspectives

From Margaret P. McLay, Chetham's, February 1991

Community music at Chetham's School of Music, Long Millgate, Manchester.

The community music project at Chetham's has been set up with the aim of showing to pupils that there is musical life outside the concert hall, and indeed that such musical activity is often vastly more rewarding. The original inspiration came from a small project some years ago which paired a group of profoundly deaf children with a partner from Chetham's. Both groups found this experience opened new dimensions for them. Further stimulation for the project came from a talk by Peter Renshaw who stressed the need to show music students that failure in a music competition did not mean failure as a musician, and that, in today's climate, musicians need to be more active in seeking out, and engaging with their audiences. The musician who is adaptable, alert and good at communicating with people, is likely to be the one who achieves a satisfactory musical career.

The Chet's course concentrates mainly on the 'non-GCSE' 4th year music group. Isabel Farrell of Live Music Now!, the music therapist Kate Fuggle, and Phil Thomas the Royal Liverpool Philharmonic Orchestra's Community and Outreach Officer, have all given talks about their work. The class has also been considering how to use their composing/arranging skills (both written and improvised) in their own performing projects, and we have also been studying performers like Evelyn Glennie, who are skilled communicators.

The class have formed themselves into duos, trios and a quartet, and chosen the type of venue in which they would like to perform. The venues chosen are: primary schools, hospitals (for the long-stay patient) and centres for the elderly. With the invaluable help of Isabel Farrell, host institutions have been sought out and I am in the process of contacting them. Pupils will have a preliminary visit to discuss repertoire this term, and next term will visit for the performance. The pupils will write a short report discussing the venue and material chosen, and assessing their own performance.

5th and 6th formers who also wish to undertake this type of project, or who wish to observe the work of a specialised music therapist, are also in the process of being accommodated.

For the future, I am investigating

1) the possibility of linking up with a small, local school for children with severe learning difficulties. Such a long–term link would allow the pupils to build up their confidence of visitng Chet's or having Chet's pupils visit them. It would allow Chet's pupils who are inhibited at working with handicapped people gradually to build up their own confidence;

2) the possibility of links with the Royal Schools for the Deaf in Cheadle where there is an excellent music teacher;

3) the possibility of an exchange–of–experience day based at Chet's for those concerned with the performing arts in the community.

In the long–run, I should like to see this work extended to all pupils at Chet's, probably in years 4 and Lower 6. I do not believe that any pupil should be forced into it, however, I hope they will quite naturally want to take part.

Comments from Chet's pupils who took part in the Community Music project performances:–

"I arranged various pieces and we announced the pieces we were going to play (which was probably the most nerve–racking part!). This arranging and announcing was new to me and I gained experience. I also learnt what was appropriate to say at the beginning of each piece."

"I have never been able to stand in front of an audience and talk about the chosen repertoire before – this was a new experience. After the first piece was performed, I began to feel very relaxed, and it was nice to be able to involve the audience. I gained a lot of confidence through this project and have never enjoyed a project so much."

"It made me research into the pieces, so I gained an understanding of the music I played."

"It was good fun."

From Richard McNicol, Apollo Trust

When the Audience Performs

Active involvement in music is central to my work as someone whose job it is to enable others to experience the fulfilment of live music-making. Nowadays my audience become fellow performers, many of them making music for the first time; music that they have invented for themselves on instruments with which they have little long-term familiarity and no specialist expertise. For me the performing process has turned full circle – if I succeed in my work, I become audience for my public.

When I decided to leave professional playing it was to develop ways of involving children of all abilities and backgrounds in live music-making. In 1977, to test the practicality of this idea, I had founded Apollo Trust. I very quickly discovered that, like me, most people love making music. The challenge was to find ways of enabling those without a "musical background" and specific musical skills to perform at a level that would give them the excitement and satisfaction with which we professional performers have long been familiar.

For me the door was opened by Peter Aston and John Paynter's wonderful book "Sound and Silence". Here was the idea that we can all be composers; that we can invent music for ourselves and, because we invent by experimenting with sounds at our own level, we are able to perform what we have invented.

This, of course, is how most of the world treats music anyway. In the West, however, a different tradition has developed. Music has become divided into categories, and composers have become associated with what many people like to call "classical" music. I had been educated to feel that it was essential to have a command of harmony and counterpoint before I could tackle the inventing of music. As a result I never got to inventing music for myself. Nobody told me that things, even then, had changed; that many composers of our time quite simply find this traditional musical language inadequate to express their musical thoughts and emotions.

A whole battery of exciting new approaches to composing have been developed, using ideas borrowed from the sounds of our modern world and transformed into musical material, mathematical and electronic sounds and a whole lot besides. These ideas offer a wealth of stimuli for our own musical creativity.

As if this were not enough, the additional stimulus of the musical vocabulary of all the peoples of the world is available on tape and disc, from Australian aboriginal music to the music of the people of Zanzibar.

I must repeat that I am not a composer. I am, however, beginning to understand how many sorts of music work and to appreciate the universality of music – that such fundamental elements as rhythm, beauty of melodic shape, colour, texture occur in all musics and excite and move us whatever their source.

I am also getting better at asking the questions and making the suggestions that enable people to release their own musicality and gain confidence in their own ideas and judgements. I am learning to help them to combine and juxtapose their ideas and above all to understand how the smallest musical germs can be developed and organised into complex and satisfying structures.

I am extremely fortunate in having continual opportunities of working in partnership with professional musicians from most of our national orchestras. My "audience" and I are endlessly excited and stimulated by the generosity with which the professionals make their performing skills available to us as a resource for our own music–making.

Still more exciting for me is to watch the musicians themselves discovering skills that perhaps they were only half–aware they possessed – skills of communication, of invention, of motivating others, and most of all, of revealing their intense sympathy for the often rudimentary early musical steps of others.

Most of our orchestras have fast–developing education and development programmes and many players reveal enviable expertise and imagination in finding their own personal ways of enabling those who would once have been mere audience to take up instruments and perform back.

By handling musical material for ourselves we gain extraordinary insight into the music of the greatest musicians of the past and of today. Throughout Britain people are being offered a new dimension to their musical experience which draws performer and audience ever closer. Many other countries are watching our revolutionary initiative with keen interest. Some have already dipped their toes into the water. Others cannot be far behind.

From Margaret Archibald, November 1991

Live Music in the Community – Its Value to the Performer

In 1989 the London Mozart Players became resident orchestra in the London Borough of Croydon. To give the full meaning to the residency the Borough was anxious to see the orchestra engaged in a wide range of community activities. Sponsorship was needed, and the orchestra was fortunate to gain the immediate and enthusiastic support of the Swiss firm Nestlé which has its British head office in central Croydon. Thus, with financial backing from Croydon and from Nestlé, topped up with an incentive award from H.M. Government, the orchestra was secure to embark on an ambitious programme of community events. Within two years more than thirty musicians, including Artistic Director Jane Glover, had engaged with a remarkably wide range of new audiences. Working mostly in small teams, musicians had provided performances and workshops for children of all ages in their own school rooms and in the concert hall, had led a regular evening institute appreciation class for adult music lovers, and had given chamber concerts for the sick and disabled in hospitals, day–centres and a hospice, with similar concerts for the elderly given in a broad range of day–care and residential institutions. The players had also provided an experimental workshop for young prisoners serving under a régime with an enlightened education policy, and thanks to a special grant from the London Borough Grants Committee had mounted a special story–time with music for under–5's which was performed in libraries. The musicians who undertook to work with these new audiences were sometimes surprised to find that they not only brought great pleasure to some of the very young, the very old or the infirm but also to themselves.

Many musicians would agree that they derive greatest pleasure from playing chamber music with others whom they like and respect. Chamber orchestras like the London Mozart Players tend to attract players who are particularly engaged in chamber music and who are therefore not only prepared to give time and commitment to community work, but who see it as an umbrella under which their existing interest in chamber music can flourish. The work requires considerable forethought, largely because the repertoire required in most community venues does not permit the indulgence of a full–scale recital of classical chamber music. Most musicians respond positively to this challenge and welcome the opportunity to extend their chamber music playing into new fields, where it is possible to include movements from favourite works but where it also becomes imperative to explore a wide range of styles. In the process each player's own musical experience is broadened and contact is made with the ethos behind music which frankly seeks to be more popular in its appeal than does most classical music.

Hitting upon a piece of music which kindles a spark of recognition in the listener so that communication suddenly takes place where there was none before is one of the rewards of this work.

The choice of appropriate repertoire is one of the most significant factors in successfully making contact with the audience. Wall-to-wall Mozart is hardly ever suitable in a community context, and it is often necessary to seek out new and unusual repertoire in order to be relevant and evocative for individual audiences. This process of discovery, whether of songs from the old days, light café music or classical chamber music for unusual but useful small combinations of instruments, can open up opportunities for players to develop their musicianship. Suitable arrangements of familiar melodies may not exist and a musician may need to make his own, or even to compose music appropriate for individual groups or for special occasions. Although the prospect may at first be daunting, it is extremely satisfying to arrange a lullaby for clarinet, horn and cello or a popular song for two violins and find that the music still communicates its essential message.

To play a wide range of music competently and stylishly requires a high degree of professionalism, and this is often more stretched in a community context than in the concert hall. The task of communicating at least something of the composer's message to each individual member of the audience in a community venue is a challenge, but it is exactly in responding to this challenge that players discover their own capacity to develop, both as musicians and as human beings. Each audience is a collection of individuals who between them have an immensely rich and varied experience of life which they can share with any musician who dares to open up a conversation with them. It can be very difficult to empathise with some groups, particularly those with learning difficulties or those who have become very withdrawn, but success in making contact on any level brings with it an enormous sense of satisfaction and achievement. The musician's job satisfaction as a cog in the wheel of an orchestra is not always very great, whereas in presenting a small-scale community concert with minimum external supervision the musician has to take the initiative and smothered creativity can be given free rein. Most of all, skills which make for more competent human beings, skills of relating to others and communicating with them, are now essential tools of the trade.

Ideally the music making, through appropriate choice of repertoire, opens up channels of communication which can then be used to develop the concert into a social occasion. The London Mozart Players use every community concert as an opportunity to socialise, so that an hour-and-a-half spent at an old peoples' home will see music being played for about half the time, the remainder of the time being spent in chatting to the residents, hopefully over a cup of tea provided by the hosts. This is especially the time when the player learns to develop sensitivity to the situation of those with whom he chats, learning to respond appropriately to people who are often seriously disadvantagd. As the musician experiences success in communicating with a wide range of people in a wide range of new ways he can only grow in confidence.

Musicians tend to work and socialise only with one another, and work in community venues enables them to meet people from a wide range of backgrounds and walks of life. This particularly includes the staff, with whom it is vital to establish a good working relationship. Hopefully these staff will come to regard the musicians as colleagues and fellow professionals, particularly if they already believe that music is intrinsically valuable. Even amongst the musicians themselves new relationships open up as they work closely with colleagues who previously had been almost strangers, in small teams in sometimes stressful situations. Thrown on their own resources with a minimum of outside interference, musicians in a small group visiting a community venue get to know one another better in a few hours than in several years of sharing the same rehearsal rooms and concert platforms as part of a large orchestra.

Despite the fact that extra preparation work is involved, one of the advantages to the player of community music–making is undoubtedly that it provides a valuable extra source of income. Many community venues are quite flexible as to when the musicians should appear and it is often possible to arrange dates so that they fit around the players' other freelance work. However, no musician who regards performing to the elderly or disabled only as something to fill the diary when nothing better is on offer should be engaged in this kind of work at all. The rewards to the musician of concert giving in the community are largely intangible and lie in the satisfaction of communicating and in the enhanced self–image which comes from believing that in the attempt to contribute to the happiness of others something worthwhile is being achieved. Above all, the community musician experiences the joy of giving and receiving, of loving and being loved.

INDEX